THE ORGAN HARVESTERS BOOK II

Other Books by Bette Golden Lamb

The Organ Harvesters

Gina Mazzio RN Medical Thriller Series (with J. J. Lamb)

Bone Dry
Sin & Bone
Bone Pit
Bone of Contention
Bone Dust
Bone Crack

Stand-alone novels (with J. J. Lamb)

Sisters In Silence
Heir Today...
The Killing Vote

The Organ Harvesters Book II

By

Bette Golden Lamb

TWO BLACK SHEEP PRODUCTIONS
NOVATO, CALIFORNIA

Dedication

**For J. J., my love, my life
and
My sons, Clifford and Michael**

Chapter 1

ORGAN HARVESTERS COMPLEX
Dissection Laboratory

They were coming.

Alarms whooped, sirens wailed, thunder boomed from the marshals' pounding boots as they ran through the laboratory from where she and her daughter had escaped from only moments ago.

Oh, my god!

Shivers of terror climbed up and down Dr. Zoe Hidalga's spine.

They would be on them in seconds.

Zoe flinched when the loud roar of the lab's ventilation fan snapped into life. She and her daughter were blasted with the biological remains of their friends, Nathan and Seka, who had been vaporized inside the lab only minutes ago.

She wanted to scream, but her throat was so laced with fear she could barely swallow. Her friends had given their lives to save her. To save her daughter, Laya.

Mother and daughter gulped for air, choked while the ashes flew from within the laboratory to where they now sat on the edge of an open vent just outside the lab. Their escape route was a drop into this huge roaring vent below their dangling feet.

Side by side, they looked down into the depths of the tube, desperate to see into a darkness that was their only exit from Emory Dutton and the Organ Harvesters.

Zoe stared into the black hole, knew it was now or never. They had to jump into that nothingness or die right here.

She picked up a loose rock from the narrow ledge and threw it down.

Silence.

"Dr. Hidalga! Stay where you are. You don't have to die. I promise that you and your daughter will not be harmed."

Emory Dutton!

His voice barked over the communication system from inside the dissection laboratory.

"Leave us alone," she shouted.

"Mommy, maybe they won't hurt us."

Zoe couldn't lie to her little girl. "They will kill us, Laya— the way they murdered Nathan and Seka."

Her daughter's eyes were huge with fear; a flood of tears ran down her cheeks.

An eight-year-old shouldn't have to worry about people killing her.

"What are we going to do, Mommy?"

Static, then Dutton's voice was screaming. "Dr. Hidalga. Come back in here now! This is your last chance!"

She squeezed Laya's arm. "We're going to jump down into this tube and when we come out we will be free from all those bad people. The ones who are trying to kill us."

One of the marshals was now on all fours, crawling through the silent disintegration chamber—a plastin oxygen mask covered his face, making him look large and alien. In a moment he would reach them. They would be trapped.

Zoe screamed and drew Laya onto her lap—they were perched as one on the edge of the abyss.

"Close your eyes, baby."

Without another word, she pushed off.

The blowing air tore at her mouth, yanked at her hair. She tried to squeeze Laya tighter, closer, but Zoe's limbs were being blasted away from her body. She could barely hold on, and then they were flung against the duct wall and her daughter was ripped from her arms.

Screams echoed all around them.

"Laaaya!"

* * *

Zoe burst out from the ventilation duct like a shot out of a cannon. Disoriented, breathless, she landed in a mountain of white ash. It blossomed all around her, closing in and choking off her air.

Frantic for oxygen, she shoved against the massive piles of human remains, holding her breath for as long as she could. Her lungs were screaming for release when she finally pushed her way out into the night. Delirious, she gasped at the low-hanging moon.

She spit out a mouthful of silty grime and tried to get some kind of foothold as she searched through the ashes.

"Laya!"

Where was her daughter?

"Laya! Where are you?"

A hand poked up through a white pile. Zoe swam through the clinging, powdery residue and grabbed onto Laya's hand, pulled as hard as she could. With no footing, she kept falling over.

Laya's face finally broke free. Her eyes were clamped shut and her mouth was filled with ashes. Zoe desperately tugged at the extended arm, searching for a solid place to stand.

It might have been minutes, or hours, before she stood on something solid.

Her daughter's face was chalky white, covered with powdery clumps of what once were body parts now morphed into ashes. No breath—not even a trace of a pulse.

She cleaned out Laya's mouth with her fingers, started forcing air down her throat, pumped at her chest, again and again. Saliva was smeared all over her daughter's face from the desperate mouth-to-mouth breathing.

Nothing.

"No! Laya! Please! We've just found each other again. Come back! Please come back to me!" She bent over and again forced air into Laya's mouth.

Her daughter suddenly sputtered and coughed, kept coughing.

"Oh, Laya. Breathe! Breathe!"

Loud rasps exploded as air pushed past the ashes in her daughter's throat. She could finally breathe.

Laya stared at Zoe for several moments." Mommy, you look like a ghost."

Zoe screamed with relief, then laughed. "So do you, baby. So do you."

Chapter 2

CEO Emory Dutton and CAPO Commander George Potek were waiting for the all-clear before entering what had become a execution chamber for Nathan Quinn and Seka Jordaine.

The Medi-Prog chief was fuming.

The fact that Zoe Hidalga and her daughter had escaped from the disintegration chamber meant little to him. Jumping down into the massive ventilation system would kill them anyway—it was a mile up from the bottom. No one could survive that fall.

Besides, Hidalga was a nobody. A diseased woman, due for termination—and that brat of hers was useless, nothing but a financial burden to the Corporits.

Nathan Quinn was another matter.

Dutton had needed him alive. Needed a firm legacy of his Corporit control. Quinn would have helped serve that purpose, even though he was a traitor to the Corporits and their way of life.

The CEO had planned a loud and disruptive trial, bringing disgrace to the Quinn family of influential doctors—doctors who wanted equal treatment for every segment of society. They had always been a roadblock to Dutton's plans and ambitions for population control with his Desisto Processing—an easy and doable mean of extermination.

Emory Dutton, CEO of the Medical Programmers, had deliberately planted Nathan Quinn in Desisto's extermination Process administration, directly under Dutton's thumb.

In that hot spot, Dutton would have made sure that the Quinns' only son would disgrace the influential family—all of them would have been brought down by simply putting a Quinn in the center of a cooked-up scandal that couldn't be erased from the family name. It was a sure way to get rid of a powerful medical group that still had enough influence to hold Dutton back. They had thwarted his goals for years.

There weren't many who could do that.

The CEO eyed Commander Potek. He stood at Dutton's side, his young, unlined face cowed.

Potek tried several times to look at Dutton, but he kept his eyes downcast. Potek had to know Nathan's death would be a big black mark on his record.

The CEO had trouble understanding the Commander. The man was in charge of the most dominating security force in the sector. He held in his fist the power of life or death, but he had no balls for a confrontation.

Coward!

Dutton chuckled to himself.

But he's my coward.

Dutton looked through the observation window into the laboratory. All biologic material had been dematerialized in the chamber at his direction.

He'd trapped the four of them—Nathan Quinn, Seka Joraine, Zoe Hidalga, and the brat—even though he only wanted Nathan Quinn. He'd wanted him alive, but push-came-to-shove, he wasn't about to let that bastard escape. Now he was dead.

The all-clear buzzer had gone off a while ago, but Dutton hadn't lived this long by taking unnecessary chances with possibly defective equipment. When he and Potek walked into the ventilated laboratory, ten minutes had passed since the all clear and he was convinced there was no chance of his being injured.

They stepped into the now spotless room. Rows upon rows of instruments used for dissection were shining as though they'd just been installed.

The marble-slab tables were sparkling, and the conveyor belt that snaked through the entire lab showed no remnants of the organs it once carried from each dissection cubicle to a massive compartment that vaporized tissue.

Even the usually preserved stacks of usable organs in holding tanks were destroyed and vented out when Dutton ordered the entire lab cleared of all biological material. That included Nathan Quinn and Seka Joraine's ashes.

"So they got away, Commander."

Potek still refused to look up. "The woman and her child are probably dead," he said, shifting from foot to foot. "That's at least something."

"Idiot! Do you think I ever cared about that diseased woman and her child?" Dutton stood up close to the Corporit Arms Protective Organizations' leader, daring him to step back and away.

Potek was too smart for that. "No, sir. I knew Nathan Quinn was our target."

Dutton pounded his fist on a nearby work table. "Then why is he dead? What good are the CAPOs if they can't bring me one person of interest—alive?"

Potek was silent.

Dutton could have sworn he'd had the Joraine woman under his control. She'd said she would do anything not to have to go back to the Vessel Procurement Center where he'd found her.

All he'd asked was that she spy on Nathan Quinn. She chose to take her chances and get into some kind of emotional entanglement. Stupid woman! Well, that didn't work out so well.

"You know, Potek, there are other protective organizations. Maybe I should think about using one of your competitors to carry out my policing orders?"

"No, sir. I think we can take care of anything you need."

It had all backfired. Dutton should never have made that traitor Chief of Desisto Processing. An idiotic mistake, but Nathan Quinn seemed so controllable.

As the head of DP, all he had to do was terminate people.

What did it matter why? Corporit leaders—the ones that really mattered—needed replacement organs. Doling them out firmly planted Dutton in charge. Where did Quinn think we were going to get the body parts we needed?

Fool!

Dutton always demanded absolute control. Every step was calculated, right down to the women he used for sex. He didn't make mistakes very often. That's how he stayed on top of the pile, how he stayed in charge of the trisector Medical Programmers in Nevada, Arizona, and California.

And he'd done it for more than thirty years.

But experience hadn't worked in his favor this time. He'd really made a mess of this. Although he would only admit it to himself, he'd horribly misjudged this whole Nathan Quinn business.

In the end it didn't matter. He would still find a way to bring the Quinns down if it was the last thing he did.

Chapter 3

NONCORP SECTOR
Care Complex #2

Godan and five of his strongest Aughts were lying in wait behind the fallen walls of what had once been a solid brick building. The ground smelled of piss and vomit.

The sun had just dropped down behind the hills—most of the day the harsh rays had been eating into his eyes; he still couldn't see shit.

Well, he knew what those three black metal giant things looked like. He'd seen them, plenty of times—even been inside a couple of them.

As his eyes adjusted to the dimmer light, he could see the waiting Noncorps spread out in every direction. They didn't look so good—coughing and spitting up the same kind of puke and foulness as Godan.

The strips of cloth the Noncorps wore weren't much better than his own rags. Their hair hung loose and grimy, wasn't even greased with animal fat and flattened to their skulls the way his was.

Dumbers. Didn't even know how to stay warm.

At least his tribe had a fire in its belly, fought every day of their lives. They didn't walk around like they were half dead, or just stand in place with their mouths half open like those stupid machines they all wanted to get into.

He heard his men yawp about the two kinds of juice they all were waiting for. One kind for the sick ones, another so they never got sick.

The wall where they were crouched wasn't too far from the beginning of the line where the Noncorps waited to walk inside the black machines.

He remembered being at a beach a long time ago, watching a wave spread into the sand. That's the way those idiots stood in the line—some spread one way, some spread close to Godan's hiding place.

Need to get the healing juice into their arms to save their pitiful lives, save them from getting sick and dropping dead. Ha! Don't matter to me whether I live or die...long as I go down top dog.

Still, he had to come.

Godan's people had been whining around the night fires, talking rebellion. He knew they would soon rise up against him if he didn't act.

Their filthy talk about bodies and brains rotting away from this VMAS crud made Godan think about doing something. And after two of the bitches he'd been fuckin' started showing him some of the purple mushy blobs on their arms, it began to really get to him.

Nasty looking things. Nothin' like he'd seen before. Just didn't look right—made even him scared.

"Now remember," Godan said, "We ain't getting any of that juice if we don't have the fingers."

"Yeah, we need to get us some more fingers," one of the men said, saliva dripping down to his chin.

Godan nodded and the five men huddled down with him.

"The last ones we had dried up, so that thing in there—" he nodded toward one of the black buildings, "ain't giving us anything without good fingers for ident. You hear?"

They all grunted.

"And no brats. Got it!"

"Why? They're easy to take down," said another with an ear torn off.

"The juice won't be strong enough for us."

"Well, you're little—you're a dwarf. You could use it," one of the others said.

"Who's the dumb shit who said that?"

No one spoke up.

"The juice won't be strong enough for me either, you stupid, mothering tit." Godan dug his pointed fingernail into the closest man, let up before he could yell out. "Pick the loners. No one's gonna lose their place to rat on us."

They all nodded.

* * *

Dusk had turned into night. The ground lights didn't reach out far enough and Godan and his men were cloaked in semi-darkness—the moon gave some light even though it barely broke through the sludge. Godan could almost feel the thick air clogging his pipes before it hit his breathers.

"I'll bust your balls if you move before I tell you," Godan said. But he knew if they didn't make their move soon, his men might run off. Godan would go back empty-handed. His tribe would be angry, rebellious. They might run away and join Tabo's followers. Godan had barely beaten his rival the last time he'd challenged Godan.

He poked his elbow twice into the man beside him, and each of the men tapped the next until they all got the signal. He reached out and yanked a Noncorp behind the wall. He sliced deeply into his victim's neck. Blood sprayed like piss in the wind. Godan rock-bashed the Noncorp's head and chopped off three fingers. Then he moved quickly into the line where the dead one had been. The others chose their own victims and did the same.

A Noncorp whined, "Hey, you weren't in line here. You trying to sneak in front of me?"

Godan pressed the point of the bloody knife against the man's balls. He backed off, making room for all five of Godan's men.

* * *

11

Godan was waiting to go inside next. He stared at the letters written on the door:

CARE
CORPORIT ANATOMICAL RESONANCE EXAMINER

"Corp'its keep the Noncorps out of Sanfrancorp by giving them healin' machines for fixin' them ... so they don't yammer at them" Godan snickered to the man behind him.

The door opened and a woman stepped out. Godan took her place inside a dimly lit chamber. He thought he remembered seeing more machinery inside, but before he could think about it a soft voice spoke: "Place the second and third fingers within the outlines of the DNA sensor."

Godan positioned the two amputated fingers.

"Thank you. Now place your third finger in the adjoining indent."

He placed the third finger and saw it being jabbed with a needle.

"Thank you. You may remove your hand."

Godan gathered the fingers as a probe moved up and down his arm, finally juicing him. It took only a minute.

"Thank you for visiting our CARE unit. Remember the Corporits have generously provided this health care for you."

The door unlatched and Godan smiled as he stepped out and one of his men took his place inside.

Chapter 4

CAPLAC DOMES

Asher Wind Storm rode the winds of the night sky. His amber eye reflected the luminescence of the earth's silvery sister moon.

Climbing, climbing. Gentle winds carried him to heights where he could see the arc of Mother Earth. The planet was suspended in a locus of emptiness.

Quiescent, silent, healing.

He dropped down, flew with the winds, searching and searching the emptiness below. Two dots of light blinked into being. They glowed from the depths of the darkness. With joy in his heart, he slid down a moonbeam, skimmed across the empty plain, and homed in on the radiance, the life essences of Zoe and Laya Hidalga.

* * *

Mother and daughter were sprawled on their backs across the piles of human ashes. Zoe stared up at the ominous Organ Harvest Complex, high and far away on a hill above them. The dim glow from the moonlight did nothing to soften the building's looming malevolence.

It was difficult to grasp that they were surrounded by thousands of incinerated body parts, transformed into massive piles of white powder—byproducts of political murders by Emory Dutton.

Zoe and Laya had escaped, but were now alone in the most desolate part of the Noncorp sector on the perimeter of Sanfrancorp.

"Mommy, what will we do?"

Zoe wrapped her arms around her daughter, wiped the loose ashes from her dark hair. "We'll rest until morning, then we'll go ... we'll go find the domes."

Zoe hugged her daughter tighter to her. Soon Laya drifted off into to an exhausted sleep. A moment later, Zoe's eyes closed.

* * *

She stood with her daughter by her side, their feet floating above the surface. Strange to be weightless, no longer rooted to the earth.

From far off, Asher Wind Storm drifted across the desolation of depleted lands. He rose up and over the mountains of ashes. Strong arms gleamed in the moonlight, stretched out and reached toward her.

His voice echoed across the emptiness surrounding her.

"Time to go, Zoe."

She clutched Laya's hand. "No, we can't leave."

Sadness kept her in this spot. From here she could look up at the death trap where her friends gave their lives so she and Laya could live. She had to stay close to the memories of those who still mattered. If the two of them left, no one would think of Seka and Nathan again—they would be lost for a second time.

Storm was at her side now. The wind became his fingers flowing through her hair. His arms encircled her, lips moved to her neck.

"Trust me, my love. Trust me."

Zoe clutched Laya as they flew through the heavens. Sparkling particles floated, blinked on and off while they whirled enclosed in a spindle of colors—red, purple, yellow—strands that bound the two of them into Storm's protective arms.

Zoe's ears were bursting with a deafening silence that yielded to the strains of mystical music—ancient harmonies reached out from everywhere and nowhere.

14

A wondrous glow shone from the moon as they tumbled through a pathway that must have existed from the beginning of time.

Silvery light shimmered on Laya's face while clusters of stars hung close by in an eerie suspension of free-form sculptures—a magnificence of brilliance in an unfolding universe.

Bette Golden Lamb

Chapter 5

THE DOMES
Arina Marek's Apartment

Zoe woke with a start, still confused by her ethereal journey with Storm. Visions of stars and spirals of nebulae had floated in and out of everywhere and nowhere. They still flashed in her head.

Had any of it been real?

The first time it had happened she'd accepted Storm and his abilities to move through time—his abilities to create, to foster life.

Why doubt him now?

Zoe stretched her legs; she was comfortable in a large bed with Laya in her arms. She squeezed her daughter. The two of them were really united.

Zoe had stayed here the first time she came to the domes. She slept in this very bed, covered by this same colorful comforter before she went back to Sanfrancorp to snatch her daughter back from the Corporit orphanage.

Had it been a week ago? Two weeks? Everything had compressed and expanded at the same time.

Was that even possible?

Although she seemed peaceful for the moment, she knew how life could turn upside down in a breath. She couldn't help but be leery. Would everything good in her life disappear again?

The Corporits had stepped in and stolen Laya when her husband Elliott died two years ago. They'd refused to give her back. If it wasn't for their close Corporit friend, Andrew Potter, Chief of Robotics, Zoe probably would have died of despair.

She eyed the purple lesions on her arms. They had been the one symptom that she couldn't ignore. She had VMAS—Viral Mal-Absorption Syndrome. She'd known she was not only sick, she was dying.

Yes, the deadly spots were now fading, but she still had VMAS floating in her blood, the same retrovirus that had destroyed her husband. She was now stabilized by a thin membranous patch on her arm. *It* had sent her into remission.

Others like her, in Sanfrancorp and around the globe, were being euthanized because they carried the VMAS virus, but she was still alive.

She'd been saved by Nathan and Seka, and Andrew Potter, who had managed to steal an active stabilizer available only to top Corporit executives.

Zoe slipped out of bed, trying not to wake Laya. She hoped that the happiness Laya would soon discover in the heart of the Noncorp center would help her find some peace. For now, Zoe would let her sleep for a little longer because when she awoke, she would remember it all—all they'd been through.

In Sanfrancorp and organ satellites across the globe, there were many thousands of huge glass tanks filled with living bodies—mostly political enemies of the corporations in power. Those victims floated in a watery world in some form of vague consciousness. They might even be fully aware that they were being devoured—slowly stripped of their body parts—bit by bit so that elite Corporits could become immortal.

Laya had seen it all.

In 2020, thirty years ago, the global corporations had taken over the planet. The bloodless revolution had given the Corporits total control. Their leaders had become murderers, performing unimaginable acts to their enemies or anyone who didn't agree with them.

Zoe looked around the room of her murdered friend, Arina Marek. She went to the wall-to-wall closet and rummaged inside, staring at all the colorful pieces of clothing that had belonged to the artist.

Most people in Sanfrancorp wore the designated uniforms of the corporations where they worked. Only the elite could wear the kind of clothes that were hanging in this closet.

Zoe searched until she found a simple pair of pants. On the shelf above she found a purple tee shirt that had a picture of an amber eye inscribed in a medallion. Most people in the Noncorp area wore the medallion to show their support of Asher Wind Storm.

The clothes she chose hung loosely—she'd lost so much weight with VMAS. Today she didn't care. She was happy. But she wouldn't allow herself to get too comfortable in her freedom.

Her friend Andrew Potter had risked his life and his whole Defy underground network to save her. She would join them in their work to not only save others, but to overturn a corporate culture that was crushing everyone everywhere.

Chapter 6

CABLE CAR CONGLOMERATE
Corporits Singles Complex #25

Pain stabbed Dr. Andrew Potter's shoulder and thigh—cut through his concentration like a laser.

He sat on the edge of his bed trying to get dressed. He had to get ready for his meeting, but the pain made him awkward and clumsy. His wounds had been filthy and infected. Now that they were healing he was a little less irritable. But they still hurt like hell.

He struggled with his pants and jiggled his leg.

"Dammit!"

He took a deep breath.

Stop complaining!

He'd been lucky. Usually any contact with the Aughts was a death sentence. He'd always made a point of avoiding the Noncorp territories where those small tribes of murderous savages camped. But Zoe needed to get away from the Corporits and the shortest route out of Sanfrancorp risked capture by the Aughts.

It seemed like only yesterday when a desperate Zoe went to a robotic diagnostic unit and the system automatically informed the Corporits she was diseased.

An immediate death sentence was issued to the CAPOs, along with the required order to capture her. If she'd been picked up, Desisto Processing would have—as with all VMAS victims—made sure she was put to death. The Corporits would waste no more time or money on Zoe Hidalga, or anyone else with VMAS.

Andrew had stepped in and helped Zoe escape the CAPOs. Together they sneaked out of Sanfancorp and headed for Asher Wind Storm's Noncorp domes, only to be attacked by Godan and his Aughts. They almost killed him. And her.

Captured, Andrew fought back and the Aughts thrust wooden stakes through his shoulder and thigh. He and Zoe both would have died horrible deaths if Asher Wind Storm hadn't rescued them.

Andrew had known Storm for many years, but he was still puzzled by Storm's ability to move through space and time. As Chief of Robotics, he was addicted to the scientific exploration and explanation of everything. Storm didn't fit into to any of the paradigms of known or theoretical science.

How did this corporal man walk a spiritual pathway in a parallel world that most could not see or imagine? One of the last Native Americans, he seemed to have access to universal information and practices that defied Andrew's understanding.

And there was little that Andrew didn't understand.

He had thought that Zoe was safe in the domes, but she'd refused to stay without her daughter. Secretly, she had returned to Sanfrancorp and, with Nathan and Seka's help, stole her daughter back from the Corporits. But the four of them ended up trapped in the Organ Harvesters complex.

He glanced at his watch, knew he was going to be late for his meeting with his Defy leaders. The fact that they met in the Robotics Surgical Theater was no accident. Being Chief of Robotic Medicine had its perks, or it used to.

The time was very near when their underground resistance group hoped to take away control from the Corporits. It was past time to bring freedom of choice back to the people on the dying planet.

Andrew carefully pulled his shirt over his head, his shoulder cried out in agony. He kept trying to ignore it. Unsuccessfully.

He never really believed Zoe and Laya or Nathan and Seka would make it out safely. Trying to get away from Emory Dutton was usually a lost cause.

And now Dutton had started looking his way. Recently, Andrew was trapped into a neural interrogation by Dutton. It had almost finished him.

He'd been lucky. Plain and simple, lucky that his Valek discipline has saved him from his brain being fried from Dutton's electronic probing. Lucky his discipline allowed him to submerge outward signs of injury to a world that watched him as though he were a bug under a microscope.

But he still hurt like hell.

Andrew continued to dress, wishing he could crawl back under the covers.

It had been a big surprise to him when Nathan Quinn went to work for Emory Dutton in the first place. But the CEO probably had Nathan in his sights right from the start. There was no doubt the big man had hoped to find something he could pin against a Quinn. It was no secret that there was a family feud between Emory Dutton and Nathan's parents, Becky and Tris Quinn.

Andrew couldn't stop thinking about the dead man.

Nathan never was a political person, never wanted anything to do with the Quinn legacy of good medicine for everyone, not just the elite. He just wanted to be left alone, do a job, and lead the good life. He had thought he could walk outside Dutton's circle and have nothing to do with all the dirty politics. But no one could afford to be indifferent. Too bad Nathan had to learn the hard way. He and Seka had paid the ultimate price for his self-deception.

Andrew's Defy underground network had informed him almost immediately that Nathan and Seka had died in the Organ Harvesters complex.

And Zoe and Laya?

23

All he knew was that they had escaped the disintegration chamber. No one knew whether she and her daughter were still alive after a suicidal jump into the massive vents.

Every time he thought about it, his heart raced. Could they drop through the ventilation tube down a mountainside and live? Could anyone?

His friend Elliott would have been very disappointed in him. Andrew hadn't taken very good care of Elliott's wife and daughter, as he promised.

Andrew continued to struggle with his clothes as though he were fighting an attacking enemy. The pain made him think again of Elliott, Zoe's dead husband.

They'd been best friends from the time they went to medical school until VMAS took Elliott's life. He remembered the last time he saw his friend alive:

Elliott had been in bed, his face pale, his body wasted. "Andrew, you're my best friend ... I trust you like no one else."

Andrew had taken his friend's hand, watched him struggle for every breath.

"I'll do anything for you."

His final words, "Take care of Zoe and Laya."

Andrew still teared up when he remembered that day. He missed his best friend, missed not only his companionship, but his advice; together they had created the Defys. And now after six years, the secret political resistance group was finally gathering momentum. Corporits had squashed individual rights and held the future of the planet in their tight little fists for the past thirty years. The Defys were determined to stop the spread of this ravenous cancer.

No more.

Elliott had died not knowing how close their rebel group was to reaching their goal. They were now on the cusp of change.

A buzz from his private telelink interrupted his thoughts. He pressed the speaker button.

24

"Dr. Potter?" Andrew recognized the voice of one of the Defys.

"Yes."

"The two docu-discs you required for your research have been added to your communicator without problem."

"Thank you." Andrew disconnected and smiled.

The coded message told him that Zoe and Laya were safe with Asher Wind Storm in the Domes.

He could breathe fully again.

* * *

Andrew stepped onto the motorized walkway that took him the few blocks to the Robotics Surgical Headquarters.

WE WILL NOT GIVE IN TO THE TERRORISTS.
VOTE!
BRING BACK THE CIC TEAM THAT HAS KEPT YOU SAFE

All the speakers around the city were blasting political propaganda the closer they got to the Corporit election.

Andrew shook his head. Pretty soon it would be unbearable.

Once inside Robotics, he headed for the decontamination entrance and presented his face for the mandatory eye scan. The vacuum seal swooshed as the door opened, and then resealed when he was inside.

In the antechamber, he stripped off his clothes and stashed them in a drawer etched with his name in bold letters. No doubt the labeling made it easier for the CAPOs to rummage through his clothes for whatever info he might be stupid enough to leave behind.

Of course, the patients who required his expertise usually were very well connected in the various corporations, or else they would have been moved on to organ harvesting. Although other methods had evolved, real organs were still the gold standard for replacement. With everyone fighting for air to

25

breathe in the limited living space, DP always finished off all the *lesser* individuals.

* * *

Pain was making it impossible for Andrew to concentrate. He knew his ex-wife would enjoy this rare moment. She always said his black ass was the most focused one on the planet. And she hadn't meant it as a compliment. She'd lashed out at him, calling him a loyal Corporit.

Well, he'd worked hard to create that illusion. He was Chief of Robotics, and had designed most of the Corporit surgical androids used not only in Sanfrancorp but across the globe. If the Corporits hadn't recognized his advanced technological abilities, he would have been trained to do something basic that was necessary only for the good of the corporations —maybe cleaning their offices.

Instead, he lived like most important Corporits, housed in a spacious apartment that had whatever he wanted or needed, while his friends Zoe, Elliott, and their daughter had been jammed into a one-room living unit—merely cogs in a wheel that made the system work.

The Corporits patted themselves on the back for their foresight to sponsor Andrew. Their wonder child had created the cybernetic CARE system. It provided healthcare to the Noncorps and was used globally as a medical handout to the shut-out masses. It not only kept them from complaining about a lack of medical attention, it held them in a life-or-death clutch.

Hiding his underground activities had been hard, but he was safe for now. But he knew luck only went so far and things were going to change if Emory Dutton caught a whiff of his opposition. And he was certainly sniffing in Potter's direction.

It was not only troubling, it was dangerous. Emory Dutton was a power-hungry bastard and Andrew needed to lie low or he could end up like his parents. They'd fought against the system, and as a result of their efforts, they were disposed of in Desisto Processing.

To the end, they were outspoken critics, refusing to be slaves to a system that put technological advancements ahead of human rights and protection of the environment

There was a time when the corporations could have saved the world from environmental disaster. Instead, they only built claustrophobic dome enclosures over the major cities to help air scubbers give urban dwellers decent air to breathe.

He remembered when there were flowers, acres of rich land with wild animals, oceans filled with sea life. But the corporations had sucked the energy from everything good or worth saving on the dying planet.

All for money. All for greed.

* * *

Andrew moved into the main decontamination chamber and held his breath. "Dr. Potter, step into the center of the area, please," the cyber voice instructed.

"Shut up, you bitch!" he yelled in the soundproofed area.

In response, a thick coat of antiseptic spray covered his entire body.

Scrub brushes began to work up and down his flesh to scourge his body of any living organisms. Most of the hair on his body had long disappeared from many years of scrubbing in these decom chambers. For some strange reason he didn't miss the hair under his arms or even on his head. But he definitely missed having pubic hair. That still looked strange, even to him.

"Lift your head, please."

"Damn it!" he screamed at the electronic voice.

The brushing fingers started at his head and entered every crack and crevice in his body. Nothing was spared, including his wounds, which were barely sealed. Each time the healing gashes were scrubbed, he bled until the process was finished.

He could usually mentally clamp down and deaden pain by using Valek's techniques of extreme-mind-overload-of-stimuli and its final release of pain. He'd been a master of the technique for most of his life. But nothing was working today.

27

The final sweep of the antimicrobial probe was fierce and exact. Each part of him had to have total clearance.

When he finally entered the surgical theater, all four men in the room turned to him.

"Sorry I'm late."

Chapter 7

NONCORP SECTOR
The Domes

Asher Wind Storm sat in the center of a large circle of fifty of his closest followers. Together with Storm, these men and women had crossed through time's galactic corridors with only one goal: To gather knowledge that would heal the dying planet Earth.

They were gathered on a hill overlooking thousands of domes that had started construction many, many years ago. Inside were remnants of a once abundant earth— vibrant forests, farms of food to feed and provide the masses.

His mother's followers, now his, had traveled across the planet for decades, helping to create self-sustaining Caplac Domes. Inside each vivarium was a mixture of plant species and life forms, all in a final, desperate attempt to save life on Earth.

Storm had carried each and every one of these acolytes to an astral realm where they were swept into a passageway beyond this galaxy. They returned altered, infused with hope to save the world.

It was to that star-filled place his mother had first taken him many decades ago when he was a child. She taught him to use his powers for the good of others, shed the false illusion that ego brings enlightenment or power.

On a glistening astral plane, Storm was directed to other essences. Invisible threads would tug and draw them together. Once interlocked, Storm was further embedded with a passion for regrowth, regeneration, revival. An unbreakable universal-spiritual bond had formed that not only lifted Storm, it helped create every new dome that rose to the sky.

* * *

Zoe watched the shimmering beams of sunlight dance over the tall redwood trees inside the massive Caplac Dome. The air was sweet, fresh. The faint sound of panpipes drifted around Zoe and Laya. It was like a storybook fairyland, so unlike the Corporit environment where they had almost been killed.

From the instant they'd entered the massive structure, Laya's mouth had remained open, showing her awe of everything she saw. Zoe laughed and watched her daughter tear off her shoes and run barefoot over the thick, green moss that covered the ground.

Laya pointed at the tallest redwood. "Mommy, that is so big." She ran her fingers across the heavy, rough bark, then danced around the tree many times before skipping back to Zoe.

Of the thousands of domes in the Noncorp zone, this was Storm's special one. It contained the geodesic shelter where he lived, studied, and meditated.

She'd been inside many of the Caplacs that covered the landscape for as far as the eye could see. Most were dedicated to raising food that fed not only the Noncorps, but the Corporits who bought their supplies from Storm.

The people who lived in the Caplacs tended to the crops. Other domes held animals or orchards, and many held varieties of plants that had disappeared across the planet.

Zoe knew these vivariums had been conceived by Storm's mother and father to protect plants in the hope that someday the protective shell could be removed. Flora and fauna would be open again to a natural environment, when humans would learn to live as one with the land.

She placed a hand on her chest where her heart warmed at the thought of Storm. She remembered being inside his home before and she'd felt calm, yet thrilled at the same time. When his arms were around her, she entered his world. A place that had brought her back to a full life with deep feeling for the first time in two years.

Storm had given her the will to live, to survive.

Yes, she had VMAS. But with the stabilizing patch and Storm's attention—could it be called medicine?—she'd grown strong again.

In the beginning she wondered who he was. Everything about him was strange. Even his name: Asher Wind Storm.

Storm?

He seemed so composed and quiet. Yet Zoe had also witnessed his passion and the turbulent power the man possessed when angered or grieved. He could turn rain to ice, travel through space, and although he belonged to this world, at the same time she knew he didn't belong. He was here ... and yet, he wasn't.

As a doctor, steeped in science, she wondered how a man could channel life to revitalize sterile soil. It looked so natural, so logical as she watched him work his magic. But at the same time it defied logic.

The answer lay hidden somewhere in the knowledge that he was the last of the full-blooded indigenous peoples who had understood the land. Somehow, Storm and his special circle of acolytes lived on a different plane of existence. Another sphere of time?

Mother and daughter walked hand in hand on the soft green moss. They soon came to a simple wooden marker. Words were scorched across the front of it:

Arina Marek
Our sister who has returned to the universe

"Is this a grave?" Laya asked, her voice solemn.

"Yes it is." Zoe smoothed Laya's stray ringlets from her eyes.

"Who is Arina Marek?"

31

Zoe crouched down so she could look into her daughter's eyes. "Arina was a great artist and friend, and very brave. You would have liked her."

"What happened to her, Mommy?"

"She was captured by the Aughts."

Laya thought a moment. "In Sanfrancorp ... in school, they talked about the Aughts. Are they really bad people?"

"I don't know." Zoe knew she shouldn't hate them, but at this moment, she did. "They killed Arina."

"Why?"

"Because. they could."

A pair of yellow birds flew to a limb above their heads and began to chirp and sing. Zoe whistled their song, the way Arina had done when she and Zoe were together. It was a wonderful memory.

Laya wandered away, but soon came running back to hide behind Zoe. The gray wolf with amber eyes stood in the pathway.

"It's okay, Laya." She pulled her daughter to her side. "That's Storm's friend, Wolf."

The animal turned, and Zoe took her daughter's hand and followed.

* * *

The wolf sat at Storm's feet. He scratched its fur and smiled at both Zoe and Laya, but his eyes only gazed at Zoe.

"Showing Laya the domes?"

"I love them," Laya said. "It's just the way Mommy said it would be. And look, the wolf has the same color eyes as yours."

"Come inside for a while," he said.

Zoe saw Laya's disappointment. "Can't I stay out here and look around?"

"Okay," Zoe said. "But don't get lost."

"Wolf will watch her." The words had barely left his mouth when the wolf walked up to Laya and stood by her side.

"What's its name?" Laya asked.

Storm laughed. "Wolf. That's what he answers to."

Laya leaped around Zoe and ran into the forest, the wolf at her heels.

* * *

Storm held out a hand for Zoe. They walked into his light-filled home.

Zoe remembered that his shelves were filled with books that would never be found in the Corporit electronic libraries. She also knew that within his home was a special laboratory, filled with microscopes and plant seedlings that he was regenerating and studying. It wasn't like any lab Zoe had ever seen.

A separate section held a greenhouse with large exotic plants that she'd also never seen before, not even in books.

"You saved us, didn't you?"

"You saved yourself, Zoe. And you saved your daughter. You were very brave." He opened his arms and she went to him.

She'd come home.

Chapter 8

Zoe loved walking Laya to school, loved the time spent in the central Noncorp community where people were spirited and friendly. Many would stop to ask their names and wanted to know all about them. When they realized Zoe and Laya were staying in Storm's dome, there was a subtle shift in attitude. Each person became more respectful. It was obvious that Storm was held in great awe—and those feelings were now spilling over onto Zoe and Laya.

At first her daughter was shy, but that changed. Now she would talk to anyone. It was easy to see her little girl was becoming happier and happier with each passing day.

Before her illness, Zoe had taken her body for granted. It was only on the brink of death that she really appreciated her health. Now with every step, Zoe knew her muscles, her whole body was growing stronger. Everything was returning to normal and she was grateful.

At the school, she watched Laya take off and play with the other students—it was as if she'd been a part of their lives forever. Her laugh rang out across the playground and it was hard to imagine that just a short time ago she'd almost died in Zoe's arms.

Laya hardly noticed Zoe slip away when the teacher took her aside.

"I think Laya is fitting right in," the teacher said. "She seems like a wonderful little girl."

"She's witnessed despicable things, things children should never have to see."

"Most of the children here have also suffered." The teacher touched her arm. "I know it's hard to let go, but it's here that she'll learn to integrate into her new life."

"I hope you're right."

"She'll be fine." The teacher walked them out of the play area. "I know you're upset about our adjustment program, but I think Laya will surprise you. When children spend the required six weeks in the dormitory, they bond very quickly and never feel alone again."

"But we've been separated for two years. We've just been reunited." Zoe looked away to hide her pain. "It's like losing her all over again."

"Dr. Hidalga, you're free to home school her if you wish ... but I think that would be a terrible mistake."

Zoe looked back at Laya. She was happy with the other children. "I'll just say goodbye to her."

She took Laya's hand and tugged her away from the others. Her daughter looked up at her with her large, dark eyes.

"Are you sure you're all right with staying here?" Zoe knew the answer *she* hoped for.

"Should I stay with you, Mommy?"

Laya was where she needed to be, that was obvious, but her little girl was willing to do whatever Zoe desired.

"No, no, I only want you to be happy."

Laya wrapped her arms around her mother's middle. "I think it'll be fun. Everyone is so nice."

"Okay, baby."

"But you'll come visit? Laya said, a worried look marring her face.

"Of course, sweetheart."

With that Zoe kissed Laya and hurried away from the school dome.

* * *

Instead of returning to Arina's apartment in the Hillsborough Mansionplex, she headed for the underground ambulated walkway to return to the metro domes.

On the way, she took more time to meander through the center of the urban Noncorp area. It was exciting to be among people who seemed so high-spirited and friendly. Everyone wore brightly colored clothes, unlike Sanfrancorp where bland corporate garb was the expected dress.

Medallions embedded with an all-seeing eye were worn by most of the people everywhere she walked. She'd never really understood the significance of the eye medallions until she saw the phenomena herself.

It was like God was in the heavens—a large amber eye watching over everyone

But it was Storm protecting them.

Storm, who wanted her near him.

Storm, who seemed more than a man, yet was only a man when he took her in his arms.

* * *

The first time she'd been in the central area, in the midst of the crowds busy shopping for food and goods, all she'd felt was alienation. She had to admit that then she'd felt superior because she was a Corporit, raised and invested in its claustrophobic lifestyle, no matter how repressive.

All that had changed.

Becoming a Noncorp meant she could practice medicine again, practice it as she first envisioned when she went to medical school. She could treat patients instead of spending her days in a laboratory dissecting organs that were torn from people who were tortured in the most unimaginable ways.

Zoe left the center of town, stepped up to the brick transportation building and placed her two fingers on the iridium plate.

The door snapped open instantly and she stepped onto an underground moving belt that carried her through the central Noncorp area to its outer reaches.

When she stepped outside of the transportation exit, wind blasted her face, coating her eyes, blinding her. While she rubbed at her eyes, someone clutched her arm.

She screamed.

Arina had been grabbed by the Aughts right here. They'd taken her away to their encampment and murdered her.

Half blind, she stumbled, struck out and freed herself, ran toward the nearest dome entrance. When her vision cleared, she saw a woman lying on the ground writhing and moaning.

"Help me." The woman looked at Zoe with pleading eyes.

She rushed back, checked to make sure there was no one else around. But it was only the woman and she was struggling to breathe. She looked up at Zoe, her eyes filled with pain. She tried to speak, but couldn't.

"I'm going to get help." Zoe saw the purple lesions on the woman's arm as she squeezed her hand. "I promise, I'll be right back."

Zoe dashed for the entrance to Storm's dome.

* * *

Storm carried the woman inside—she died in his arms. He set her down on the soft, mossy ground. "I'm sorry. She's gone."

"No! She was still breathing when I found her." Zoe moved in close and tried to force air into the woman's mouth, compressed her chest. Storm placed a hand on Zoe's shoulder.

"She's gone."

But Zoe kept working frantically until he set both hands on hers.

She looked down at the woman's distorted face, her clothes, really only shredded rags knotted together; they barely covered her filthy body. Every inch of her was caked with dirt that had been a part of her skin for a long time.

She held up the woman's arm to display the spread of the rampant purple lesions. "She was too far gone."

Storm nodded.

"She looks like an Aught."

"Yes. She is."

"Why was she out there alone?"

"People who have been given the tainted VMAS stabilizer have been dying all over the globe." Storm nodded to several men who had arrived to help. They lifted the dead woman and carried her away.

"But why wasn't she with her people?"

"She was young, probably ran away to get help."

"Everyone seems unaffected in this part of the Noncorp area," Zoe said. "Why haven't your people died?"

"We found out about the Corporit lie when Andrew Potter sent us the real stabilizing membrane. One like yours, not the one that murders people."

He held her hand and they walked through the trees. Soon Wolf materialized out of nowhere and moved to Storm's side.

"And the Aughts?"

"Some tried to help themselves. They thought they were getting vaccinated when they went to the CARE centers. But like everyone else, those who were already infected have been dying like that woman."

Zoe was agitated. She'd seen what Storm could do to help others and he'd done nothing.

What was the matter with him?

She could hear the anger in her own voice. "Why aren't *you* helping the Aughts?"

"You don't understand."

"Well, help me to understand. You have tremendous powers, Storm. You float with the wind, see everything. How can you ignore those people?"

A flash of anger crossed his face, gone before it could imprint his features. When he spoke it was with a detachment that did nothing to make Zoe feel better.

"All is chosen, Zoe. Godan, Tabo live by their own rules. The Aught tribes don't want anyone interfering in their way of life."

"I don't believe that. You said Aughts went to the CARE center, and that woman who just died wanted someone to save her. That's why she came here. She wanted to live. Why can't we make sure everyone is vaccinated? Everyone should receive the real stabilizer. At least if we can't save them, we can help them die peacefully."

"You didn't feel that way when they murdered Arina, or when they almost killed you and Andrew." His eyes seemed to burn through her.

"You're right," she said. "Then I was thinking like a victim ... not a doctor."

* * *

Zoe and Storm had eaten a dinner of wild mushrooms mixed with sprouts and eggs, and a vegetable soup that was so delicious she'd had a second bowl. They talked about Laya and her new school.

Zoe was already lonely for her daughter, but it was the death of the Aught woman that made her feel powerless. Storm picked up his panpipe and began to play; it put her into a meditative state—the music was haunting, filled with melancholy yesterdays.

Memories of her former life still lived in her heart. It would be hard to become a Noncorp when she'd always been a Corporit—yet it was beginning to feel a lifetime ago.

The soft melodious music reached for her. It cut through thoughts of her uncertain future.

Wolf lay down at her side; she ran her fingers through its fur. Every now and then it would look up at Storm and then at her. Twin sets of amber eyes would then turn to her.

Storm lay the pipes down, opened his arms, and she folded into him as if she were born to be there.

"I have to go, Storm."

"I know."

"I can't ignore it. I have to do something to help those people. No one else is." She looked up at him. "Do you understand?"

"Of course." He pulled her closer, his fingers pressing her to him. "Once I felt as you do. And because of that we've brought many of the Aughts into our population. They are now free to join us at any time. Most have. Godan and Tabo have always resisted. Godan murders for the pleasure of killing."

"Do you really think he would kill me for trying to help his people?"

"I don't know. What I do know... I can't lose you."

He squeezed her even tighter and she was enveloped by all of him, caught up in a wilderness of sensations—the smell of his hair, his skin. When she closed her eyes, she was reborn among fields of flowers, trees, and the earth, wandering in a world she remembered as a little girl.

But with his arms around her, she also remembered what it was like to be a woman.

Chapter 9

Asher Wind Storm spun into a whirl of dust that tossed over the land. He twirled around and around and around until his rational self surrendered to the wind.

Free, free, free.

He lifted higher, higher into the layers of air where momentum carried him until the domes were far below.

The Caplac Domes were still spreading across the earth filled with plants, with animals, with life. He hoped their future would be to reclaim and regenerate the Earth. Bring back a time when the domes could be cast aside.

Soon the sight of land was gone and he was again lifted until he pierced the upper stratosphere. There he was beyond the polluted atmosphere surrounding the planet.

At last he could see the stars and his sister moon. Out here there was a different kind of life—everything thrived in universal splendor without the distortion of the planet's decay.

This was where he went to find the spirits of the wise ones. The wellspring of his revelations.

The moon called to him, as it had so many times in the past. Its soundless vibrations flooded him.

What was its message?

What was its secret, waiting for him to grasp?

He held his arms out, closed his eyes and surrendered his soul to the everything. Floating, floating, waiting to be suffused with the wisdom of the universal wise ones.

A microsec of infinity passed and images raced through him: Pristine waters, wild forests, sweet, pure air.

Memories crowded his mind, each rivaling the other.

But one image remained the clearest.

Our Mother Earth still struggling against the final throes of existence.

Sudden anger shook him. The anger he had always had to control to keep himself clear from human taint——it always craved revenge and it bred hatred. If he relented his mission would be lost.

His mission?

Save our Mother. Save our Mother Earth.

* * *

Godan sat on his rock high above the encampment. This was his kingdom. He was born into it and it was all he had ever known. Here was the place where his power rested. Where his future lay.

But he was tired. So tired.

Two of the women he'd slept with had died. Two days ago his children had also died.

He picked at a pustule at the tip of his nose. Many were erupting all over his body. The pain was beyond unbearable; it blinded him with flashes of red and orange hell. Even when he withdrew his pointed nail from the point of decay, the intensity continued.

He stood and screamed, shaking his fist at the sky.

There is no great one. My father lied. There is no one.

A string of violent coughs racked his body. He couldn't breathe until he coughed up clumps of blood-soaked rot. His legs became weak and felt like water. They would not hold him.

He sat.

When would his chest stop burning? When would the ripple of uncontrollable shivers stop tearing at his body every single night? What if this weakness never ended? Or became worse?

Half of his followers were dead. They had dropped to the ground, spilling their guts, dying where they fell, their bodies covered in purple mushy things.

Would this have happened if they hadn't gone to the healing machines at the edge of the Noncorp territories? He

44

thought the juice squirted inside and the patches on their arms would save them from dying. That's what was said, why they went there. But now he knew the truth—every single person who wore the patch was dead.

It was his fault. All because he had agreed to get the medicine. Somehow, everyone had been tricked. Rumors said Corp'its had been tricked, too. He should never have believed the Corp'it words.

He lay down on the ground in agony and closed his eyes.

* * *

From far away, Godan heard the alarm, but he was too tired to move or even care. When he rolled over, he looked into the stony eyes of his rival tribal leader, Tabo. Instead of jumping to his feet ready to fight to the death, Godan didn't care.

He turned his head away. This time was as good as any to die.

The dwarf lay there in silence, waiting. And when the moments passed and he was still alive, he turned back to his rival and looked hard at him.

Tabo is sick and his men look as weak and as puny as mine

The excitement Godan should have felt wasn't there. He'd hated Tabo since they were children. It was said they shared the same father, but when Godan had threatened to kill his mother if she was silent, she denied they were brothers.

He didn't believe her.

Tabo held out a hand. "Let me help you."

"Kill me and get it over with, you bastard."

Tabo pushed his hand out farther. "I want to talk."

He held onto Tabo and allowed him to pull until he was in a sitting position. Then Godan stood upright.

"My people are dying." Tabo pulled a knife sheathed in his waistband and threw it on the ground. "Everything is changing."

Godan withdrew his weapon from its sheath. "That was a mistake, Tabo ... you don't make many of them."

Tabo showed no fear.

45

"It's time to leave the garbage pits. Come to the domes with me, Godan. Come if you want you and your followers to survive."

The dwarf looked down upon the encampment. His people were moving around, but they were walking like mindless human shells. Even the few children were like slugs, lifeless.

Godan's spine stiffened. "You want to take my tribal land from me. You want control of my Aughts." He stared back at Tabo, who had lost an eye since they last fought and new scars crisscrossed his face. "Well, you can't have them! Not without a fight."

Three of Godan's best men had scrambled up to the towering rock. They silently moved to his side.

"Haven't you lost enough? And still you live in the Corp'it waste pits."

Tabo spoke in a voice that Godan had never heard. Strong, but with the sound of truth that made Godan hesitate.

This is a trick. Tabo can't be trusted.

Godan felt his strength returning. "Leave now or fight!"

Tabo looked strangely at Godan. Before the dwarf could react, he snatched up his knife from the ground and placed it back into his waistband.

"Remember this day, Godan. There will not be many more left for you and your people."

In the blink of an eye, he and his men were gone.

Chapter 10

SANFRANCORP
Medi-Corp offices

Dutton was still ignoring his telelink. It had been buzzing and blinking nonstop ever since he walked into his penthouse office at 9:00 AM.

At this hour, he liked to walk at a leisurely pace to his window in the tallest building in the city, look down on everything from the top of his world. Coffee in hand, he would study the intricate array of the many architectural patterns before he settled down to start work.

Each day he made it a point to study the dome that covered all of the new Sanfrancorp city limits, hoping it was still holding up, not cracking open as it had been projected to do almost from the time it was completed. Without that amber covering, they'd all be sucking filth and carbon into their lungs.

It was reassuring to know that Chemcorp was working on a potential gel of some sort to fill in and seal any imperfections or cracks that might develop. Dutton thought Chemcorp was a solid company with fine leadership and he was confident it would solve any possible problems concerning the dome's integrity. After all, the company had been an excellent investment for him and he refused to worry about it. But he still compulsively checked on it every day.

Today, he was too agitated to stand at the window and stare out into space. The worst part was having to listen to the constant roar of political announcements, backing the Corporit chosen candidates for the powerful Corporit International

47

Council. They'd been blasting on and off throughout the city all day.

Instead, he sat down at his desk and watched split-screen images of cities around the world and their response to the VMAS accelerator killing off infected people. From what he could see, Moscowcorp was the most violent, with Londoncorp next in line.

Reports were coming in from everywhere. Right now local shots of Sanfrancorp mobs filled his screen as people tried to knock down the CAPOs. He had to admit there was a lot more rioting than he'd bargained for.

With all the unwanted attention being heaped on him since they'd made the VMAS stabilizer lethal, he'd had to take sleeping medication just to get the rest he needed—and his sex life, which he always liked to brag about, was nonexistent.

Communications were flying back and forth with messages from the CEOs of corporations within Emory Dutton's tristate district—from the shoe manufacturer to the pharma bigwigs—and he knew he would also be hearing from Corporits from all over the globe.

He'd refused to answer any calls on his telelink for the last several hours. He knew what it was about—everyone was alarmed and angry and wanted answers. He could imagine what was going on in their heads if they all had followed his advice for vaccination and stabilization of VMAS.

He turned back to the nonstop blink of the telelink.

Complain, complain. Complain about the crowding, lack of food, lack of work, but the minute you do something constructive about it, they chicken out.

Well, nobody liked reality, but that's where the solutions lay. Either cut the population numbers or we're all going down.

You can't make and omelet without breaking eggs.

Even he'd begun to notice how much he used that hackneyed phrase. And he'd caught some of his staff rolling their eyes when he used it.

His new assistant, Astrid, came into his office without knocking.

"Sir, News-Div refuses to take no for an answer. They're in the waiting room insisting on an interview now."

"Tell them to wait. I'll talk to them when I'm good and ready."

"Sir—"

"You heard me. Now get out!"

He knew he'd hired her for her well-shaped ass as much as anything else, but he'd lost any interest today. He had no desire to watch her wiggle out of his office. Instead, he thought about her name and all the biblical names that so many people had today. For some reason those names spoke to him of pending doom as much as anything that was bound to happen.

I must be losing it thinking about a stupid non sequitur at a time like this.

He hit the interoffice communication line. "Astrid, get Potek in here. And don't let him give you any excuses. Tell him I want him here now."

He clicked off before she could reply and turned back to the live video feed and population communications citywide. The screen was filled with scenes of streets covered with masses of bodies sprawled everywhere. Many shots showed bulldozers lifting clots of bodies being carried away for massive burial.

I've really fucked up. Never dreamed there were so many people infected with VMAS in the city.

He turned back to the nonstop flashes on his telelink, then immediately looked away.

Astrid stuck her head in the door. "Commander Potek is here, sir."

"It's about time."

* * *

Commander George Potek could see from the look on Dutton's face that this was not going to be pretty.

49

He was used to the CEO's tantrums and he kept body and soul together by telling himself that one day he was going to punch him out—maybe even kill the bastard. Even though it was only a fantasy, it got him through many a dress-down.

But the facts were the facts.

Without Dutton's Medi-Progs, Potek's company was going down. He would be finished.

"Do you see what's going on out there?" Dutton pointed to the flashing scenes scrolling across his communications screen. "What are you doing about this?"

"Our CAPOs are out there trying to maintain order."

"Is that a fact?" Dutton nodded at one screen where the mob was turning really ugly, pushing back hard at the marshals, who were tasering so many people you could see the sparks flying everywhere.

Potek's stomach was flipping and he was swallowing so hard he could barely speak. "Trust me, when we get the bodies off the streets, things will quiet down, sir."

"Trust you? Isn't that what I always do?"

"Sorry, sir ... what I meant is, it will return to normal as soon as we can clear the streets of the corpses."

Dutton was pacing in circles around him.

Potek wanted to be anyplace but here. "I was thinking—"

"Oh, that would be something." Dutton kept circling him. Potek could feel nervous sweat rolling down the back of his neck. "I saw News-Div in the reception area ... I thought maybe if we could blast a news bulletin confirming that the Aughts and Noncorps have joined forces—"

Dutton stopped in his tracks. "Terrorists! Of course. Aren't they responsible for anything that goes wrong? Blaming them won't do much for the eyewitnesses, but if we hit the public with twenty-four-hour propaganda it will work. It always does. Potek, I should have thought of that sooner."

Yeah, sure, you should have.

Dutton patted Potek on the back and he could finally breathe again. The CEO stopped huffing and puffing his dragon fire around him, went to his desk seat, and collapsed into it.

Dutton pushed the button for his interoffice communicator. "Astrid, tell the News-Div people I'll be out with a statement presently."

"Yes, sir."

"Before I do that interview, bring me a fresh cup of coffee with a piece of coffee cake. And warm it up."

"Coming right up, sir."

Emory Dutton took a deep breath, leaned all the way back in his chair, then smiled.

Potek merely nodded.

* * *

The minute Dutton stepped into the reception area, reporters for all the electronic outlets of News-Div rushed in and crowded around him. Cameras began recording the session.

One of the news staff shouted, "Mr. Dutton, the city is drowning in dead VMAS victims. Did you anticipate this extensive catastrophe?"

Dutton raised a hand and scowled at the man who asked the dumb question

"I will make a statement and there will be no questions."

The room quieted. Dutton made them wait while he drew out the moment.

"Some of the people who have died on the streets of Sanfrancorp have indeed been VMAS victims. But the majority are victims of a far greater threat than any disease."

Another reporter jumped in. "Wasn't the stabilizer supposed to stop the progression of VMAS?"

"I said I would make a statement and there would be no questions." Dutton pointed at the man. "What's your name?"

"Ethan Taylor."

"Well, Mr. Taylor, you can see yourself out the door right now."

"But—"

"Do I have to call security?"

As the man went through the office door, Dutton said, "Since the question is hanging in the air, I will answer it. The stabilizer was not effective on all people, so some have died, a natural outcome of their diagnosis."

Dutton took the moment to walk back and forth in front of the reporters until he gathered their complete attention again.

"Most of the deaths are a result of a massive attack by the Aughts and many of their allies in the Noncorp community. Plain and simple, Sanfrancorp has been under attack by terrorists. As always, we will protect our own."

All the reporters' hands shot into the air.

"I'm not taking questions at this time. I thought I made myself perfectly clear about that."

Dutton looked every News-Div reporter in the eye.

"And that is all I have to say."

Chapter 11

SANFRANCORP
News-Div Bullpen

Jin Bacha sat at the computer keyboard, fingers pounding out copy for the citywide communication feeds. She was the only one who was busy. The other reporters were sitting around shooting the breeze about the bullshit CEO Emory Dutton had tossed at them earlier. Jin was having trouble concentrating, but it was an easy assignment so she only half-listened to them gripe.

"That Dutton's an ass!" Ethan Taylor said, still miffed at having been thrown out of the press conference.

"What did you expect?" Will Pronhack, his close buddy, said, reaching for a doughnut from a large platter an assistant had just brought in. "The man rules with an iron fist."

One of the others piped in, "And you, Ethan Taylor, defender of the truth, always have to push things to the limit."

"Shit, aren't we supposed to be reporters? I'm tired of being the only voice of sanity around here. For god's sake, don't you think it's time we stopped brown-nosing every CEO we interview?"

"We're just trying to hold onto our necks—you're a shit-kicker," Will shot back.

Everyone laughed, but it was an uncomfortable ripple that had nothing to do with humor.

Jin had never realized how much News-Div lied to the public until she became a Corporit reporter. It blew her mind that the news organization she'd looked to for some kind of truth was only a tool of the elite.

As a junior staff member, she barely hung onto the lowest rung of the ladder. She was supposed to be a journalist, but she spent most of her time running errands and formatting dictated copy for the streaming newsfeeds that never stopped running.

The copy was hand-delivered to her and she made sure a continuous flow of information made it to a lighted strip at the top of every building in the city. It was supposed to keep everyone informed. And it informed everyone with what News-Div wanted the public to know.

Still, Jin knew being a junior press corp member had some advantages.

Because she was a nobody, she was of no interest to this bunch or anyone else. No one paid much attention to her with her average-looking straight hair and brown eyes. She wasn't pretty enough to warrant anybody's attention. Sometimes she felt almost invisible.

And that was a good thing.

When people used to fawn over her it was only because she was a Quinn. They never really looked at *her.* All they cared about was her name. So she'd dropped her maiden name the minute she got married five years ago—now she only used her husband Melik's family name, Bacha.

Still, if anyone really bothered to dig into her roots, they would find that Nathan Quinn, recently murdered in the Organ Harvester's complex, was her cousin. And his parents, Tris and Becky Quinn, were her aunt and uncle.

She'd been very close to Nathan. After he died, she spent two days in the bathroom, crying on and off, swearing that she'd find a way to avenge her favorite cousin's murder.

Murdered by Dutton's Medi-Prog Corporation.

Her mind drifted off and she thought about her husband. Until recently, Jin thought she loved him, at least cared about him. But he saw nothing wrong with the Corporits being a privileged group that ruled the world. And the way he talked about the average person made her skin crawl.

Yes, things were just fine the way they were, according to Melik.

Of course, he *would* feel that way.

The Bacha family held a majority of the stock in Instrucorp, the corporation that supplied dissection instruments for the Medi-Progs and its Organ Harvesters outlet. Their huge, thriving business guaranteed that Melik wouldn't appreciate her and the Quinn family's radical ideas. And he let her know that in no uncertain terms after they got married. So she kept her thoughts to herself. The less he knew, the better.

She finished polishing her latest bulletins based on the Dutton interview and in a moment that blast of news would race across the city.

Aughts Join Forces with Noncorps
Murderous Rage Shakes Sanfrancorp
Bodies Pile Up Around The City

Jin sat back in her seat, her finger poised over the send button.

Lying murderous bastards! Do you think this will cover up the truth?

As she pressed the send button, a loud noise startled her.

The door to their news offices burst open and ten CAPOs stomped by her, filling the area with the smell of gun oil. They marched up to Ethan, their helmets hiding their faces.

"Are you Ethan Taylor?" The leader reached out and yanked hard at Ethan's arm. The others reporters backed away to the other end of the room.

"Ease up, man! It's pretty obvious you already know damn well who I am."

The CAPO slapped Ethan hard across the mouth. "One more word out of that mouth of yours and I will taser you with enough volts to kill you. Am I making myself clear?"

Ethan nodded, but he still had a defiant set to his mouth.

Jin sat on her trembling hands and watched Ethan walk out, surrounded by the marshals.

Chapter 12

MEDICAL PROGRAMMING CORPORATION
CEO Office Suite

Emory Dutton sat at his desk tapping his fingers. Sitting across from him was the arrogant reporter who'd had the nerve to challenge him at the news conference. A defiant look was smeared across his face.

Still living in the past when journalists had some clout, when people even bothered to listen to them. Well, those days are long gone, Mr. Reporter.

"Now what was the question you seemed to think was so important that you had to interrupt my news conference?"

The reporter didn't answer right away. He just sat there glaring at Dutton, looking like he was going to launch an across-the-desk attack at any moment. When Ethan Taylor did speak, the words came out in a rush.

"Why isn't the stabilizer working to stop the VMAS symptoms? You're blaming all those dead bodies on terrorists." He sneered. "I don't think so, Mr. Dutton. You lied. Why?"

"I suppose you expect me to answer that?"

Ethan nodded.

"And, no doubt, you intend to continue asking that same question over and over until you get an answer?"

"Damn right."

"You're sure you won't change your mind, Mr. Taylor? Think about it for a moment. I've always had a great deal of respect for the power of the press, which is why I'm asking if you can bite down on that tongue of yours, shut your mouth, and let it go. We can work together. News-Div has been good about cooperating ... until today."

"People have a right to know the truth."

Dutton picked up a pencil. First he tapped the point on the desk, then he flipped it and tapped the eraser.

"You do know the planet is dying, Mr. Taylor—"

"That's—"

"Don't interrupt me." Dutton carefully put the pencil down in front of him. "We have too many people on this planet, and not enough of anything to maintain them ... if we are going to survive we have to cut the population."

The reporter was silent.

"The VMAS stabilizer was enhanced with a virus that would terminate whoever used it within three days."

"That's murder! How could you possibly do that?"

"How could we *not* do it?" Dutton laughed. "You haven't understood a word I've said, have you?"

Dutton picked up his telelink and spoke into it. In a moment his assistant opened the door.

"What can I do, sir."

"Get Potek on the line."

* * *

Four marshals hurried Ethan towards a van —on the side was printed in bold. dark letters:

CORPORIT AIMS PROTECTIVE ORGANIZATION

The CAPOs were rough, taking every opportunity to push him with their long wooden batons if he didn't walk fast enough. He was shoved hard into a seat, with a CAPO on either side of him.

Okay. You're CAPOs. We all know you have to be tough.

He didn't mind. Let them do their thing. He felt pretty good about standing up to Emory Dutton. You couldn't be a good journalist and cower.

58

Even CEOs need to hear the truth.

He thought they were taking him back to the News-Div offices, but after a few minutes he could see they were leaving the center of town and heading towards the outskirts.

Shit, they're going to toss me into the Noncorp zone.

He tried to quiet his mind, but his stomach was going into spasms and his heart was racing so fast he could barely breathe.

Then he recognized the Nicola Fountain Sculpture. He'd been there a couple of years before when he wrote a story about Sanfrancorp's few remaining fountains that still used running water. It was one of the really beautiful ones.

They pulled up to a huge, gray complex. A large sign in front said:

ORGAN HARVESTERS

He'd barely noticed the facility the first and only other time he'd been in this area. Now, he saw it looked more like a prison. Windowless, menacing, ugly.

"Get out!" A female CAPO jammed him hard in the ribs.

"Okay. You don't have to be so rough."

"You don't know what rough is, buddy." She poked him again and laughed.

There was no reception area inside the entrance, just dark hallways. They pulled him along to a door marked:

Preliminary Workup

Ethan's mind went numb. He could hardly speak the words, "What am I doing here?"

The CAPOs laughed as though it was the funniest thing they'd ever heard, but a waiting team of three men, dressed in white coveralls, were not laughing.

One of the three said, "Strip him down!"

"No!" Ethan turned and tried to run. "Stop! There must be some mistake."

One of the CAPOS poked him back toward the team. "There's no mistake, big shot."

"Careful with those weapons," the tallest team member said. "Don't damage the goods."

Ethan started screaming. His loud cries pierced the air. "Help! Help me!"

The tallest man in white said, "Fuck Dutton! Give him a sedative. I can't work with all those screams."

Ethan watched one of them grab a syringe and a rubber tourniquet.

"Now don't fight me, 'cause this will help you get through it. Hear me?"

Ethan nodded.

He was naked. His head was spinning when they laid him down on a table. He became an observer, watching everyone move around him.

One of the CAPOs yelled out, "Goodbye, sucker."

The words didn't mean much to him.

The tall man in white seemed to be in charge, but Ethan turned and stared up into the blinding lights over his head.

The leader said, "Let's get this done with. We have a whole stack to tackle today."

They spent a long time washing his belly and cleaning his mouth with burning solutions. He was starting to doze off when a stabbing pain cut through him. "Oh, my god, that hurts." The words were clear in his head but they came out in a garble. He looked down and saw a large tube sticking out of his middle.

"I'm not going to kid you, man. The rest is going to be pure hell."

The leader jammed a tube into his mouth and down his throat. His lungs were on fire.

Stop! Please stop! Stop! Stop!

Chapter 13

SANFRANCORP
Cable Car District

Tris Quinn grabbed his wife Becky's arm and they shoved their way through large clots of screaming people. Adults and children were crashing to the sidewalk—mouths foaming, arms and legs thrashing.

Tris watched in horror; they were in a vortex of falling bodies that spun all around the two of them.

Nathan had warned this would happen before he died. He'd come to Tris to get the real stabilizer, the ones they used to save the CEOs—he needed it for his friend, Zoe Hidalga.

The new vaccine for VMAS had been given to all populations. Uninfected people would have permanent protection, but infected people were getting a transdermal accelerator. The small skin patch was killing anyone with the retroviral organism in their system.

Tris learned that the CARE units in the Noncorp zone had been supplied the week before. Today was the third day since the new Corporit mass vaccination.

And this was the result.

It was happening everywhere, in every Corporit city across the globe, killing thousands upon thousands of people.

The thought of Nathan made Tris's breath catch, made him wish he were dead instead of his son.

His only child was gone and all he wanted to do was lie down and die, sprawl next to all the bodies on the sidewalk; let them carry him away. That would end the hollowness that drove him to despair each and every day from the moment he opened his eyes. But he couldn't do that to Becky. She would grow to hate him, to hate his memory for leaving her alone to face a world without Nathan.

* * *

Becky knew Emory Dutton had lied to the medical staffs to get their cooperation. Only the chiefs knew about the deception, and they were threatened with expulsion to the Noncorps if they didn't follow orders.

They'd had to keep the secret.

Instead of advocates for patients, doctors had become babes on the corporit tit. They had to do what they were told.

Becky Quinn could still remember when doctors protected their patients. That was before corporations started pulling the strings. Now, medicine was just another business, another arm of the Corporit structure.

She watched the squadrons of CAPOs arrive to this scene out of Dante's *Inferno*. Becky clutched Tris's hand and tears ran down her face as they shoved their way out of the center of the mob to a storefront. At least they were at the edge, out of the worst of it. The CAPOs were shoving, stick-beating, tasering anyone close to them who was still standing, or who wouldn't settle down. Then they dragged the troublemakers away in vans. They would be taken to prison and who knew what kind of torture they would receive there?

The two of them held onto each other's hands, stepped over the dead bodies that would soon be hauled outside the city's covering dome and cremated in huge bonfires. The stink of death would be around for weeks.

"We could have saved these people," Tris said. "They could have had the real stabilizer, the way Zoe did."

"No time for that now, Tris." Becky tugged at his arm. "We have to get to the hospital. They're probably being swamped with trauma injuries from mob-panic or the CAPOs going crazy."

She could see Tris didn't want to go. He wanted to go home.

"I can't do this."

"Tristan Quinn! Don't you dare back out. We're doctors. We have to help. Do what we can. Do you understand?"

"I don't want to, Becky."

She turned his head, stared hard at him. "You have to do this, if for no other reason than Nathan would have wanted you to."

She looked into his dark eyes, saw the young, fiery man she'd fallen in love with. That man would never have said no to helping people.

"We're going to get that bastard Dutton if it's the last thing we do." She clutched his arm. "Do you hear me?"

After a long moment, he said, "I do!"

* * *

CABLE CAR DISTRICT 3
Corporit Hospital

When Tris and Becky arrived at the hospital, they stood dumbstruck.

Tris looked at the walls and floors covered in blood splatter. Everyone stood in coalescing globs of it, slipping and sliding in the viscous mess, trying to keep from falling down.

Administration had expanded the ER. There were tents outside the hospital walls and the ER had taken over the hallways of other service areas.

Everything had been turned around. Under normal circumstances, the emergency room was very small. Most patients the regular staff treated were from wealthy families. The rest of the populace fell into three categories and dispensed with very quickly:

Come & Go, Selective Euthanasia, Organ Harvesters.

Today, Tris and Becky were among only a handful of doctors who had come to help in this writhing snake pit filled with human flesh.

People pushed others out of their way to get medical attention. Some of the doctors and nurses were threatened with knives. There was a roar of voices.

"They just suddenly fell, clawing at themselves!" one woman screamed over and over.

A pregnant woman shrieked, "They stabbed my husband." She held out her arm. "Look what they did to me." Blood was dripping from a gaping wound.

A chorus of people were yelling the same time: "Help me!"

A man with vacant eyes said, "They all started pushing, running. The mob became an avalanche, trampling kids, crushing everybody."

The noise was unrelenting. Women screamed, pulled at their hair; men shrieked and cursed god.

Mothers and fathers walked in a trance, carrying their broken, dead children, begging the medical staff to bring them back to life. There were masses of people with penetrating, slashes across their guts—terrified people had cut and sliced at themselves, screaming about devils. They walked in tight circles as they tried to stuff their insides back into their bodies.

Becky knew what Tris was thinking. She wanted to run away, too.

Chapter 14

Robotics Unit

Andrew Potter was coming back from lunch when he looked up at the headline on the closest building.

Aughts Join Forces with Noncorps ...
Murderous Rage Shakes Sanfrancorp
... Bodies Pile Up Around The City

Son of a bitch! That goddam Dutton. I should have seen this coming. He's never going to take any responsibility for this mess.

Except for the CAPOs and security vans, it was rare to see automotive vehicles in the city, much less trucks. Today monster semis were everywhere.

Like stacked steel beams, bodies were neatly piled on the side of the streets, ready to be set inside the carriers and taken away.

Potter knew the deal The bodies would be quickly removed, taken out of sight to quiet the agitated population—then the people would do whatever they were told to keep the terrorists away.

He hurried into the Robotics Unit and rushed to his office. When he walked onto his wing he stared at the woman at the reception desk. He'd never seen her before.

Ignoring her, he walked into his office. An unknown assistant was straightening his desk.

"Who are you?"

"Good afternoon, Dr. Potter. I'm Regina, your new assistant."

"Wait a minute! I didn't request a new staff member. What was wrong with my last assistant? Where is she?"

"I don't know, Doctor. I was told to report this morning. So here I am." She was very young and pretty. She gave him a wide smile, tried to perform a low curtsy, but she almost fell over. He reached out to steady her, catching a whiff of some kind of perfume.

"What happened to Anya?"

"As I said ... I don't know."

"Why do we have a new waiting room receptionist?"

Andrew Potter now knew he would be under constant surveillance by Dutton. This was really going to make things difficult.

"I can try to find out."

He gave Regina a forced smile. "Forget it."

Andrew went to his computer and created a long list of schematic files the new assistant would have to bring up and pore over for the information he was requesting. They would be difficult to find and differentiate. She would be at it for hours.

"I've just sent you a list of files that will need to be collated, and reclassified, according to disease."

"I'll get to it right away."

He again smiled at her. "Close the door when you leave, please."

When she left, he let the mask drop away.

It's past time for the Defys to take real risks. Time to move to Plan B.

* * *

Dutton was sitting across from Maxwell Morgenthau in The Upper Crust, a posh restaurant that required CEO status for membership. Not a very original name for an exclusive establishment, but it said what had to be said about who was going to be allowed to join.

The CEO of News-Corp sat at table strictly reserved for Dutton. Everything was crisp and fresh. Repli-roses in a cut crystal vase sat in the middle of the table, the petals as real as any Dutton remembered from long ago. His spot was surrounded with simulated waterfalls. The piped-in sound of the water always relaxed him.

When Dutton sipped his martini, M.M. stared at his tall glass of water, and gulped down a large swallow.

"Not drinking, I see."

M.M. only nodded.

Dutton laughed. "Well, you do look a little yellow around the gills. Something wrong?"

"I need a new liver," M.M. said, his voice choking up. "If I don't get one soon ... I'm going to die."

"Didn't we just get you one of those a year ago?"

M.M. nodded. Took another huge gulp of water.

"I remember you got that prime piece of meat from a beautiful young woman." Dutton ran a finger over the lip of his martini glass. It made a small squeak. "An uncooperative beautiful young woman." He laughed. "One who wouldn't toe the line. You know how it is. They either give in or they become prime donors, like it or not. Good looks only buy you so much slack."

M.M. nodded again.

"So you drank through that one, too."

M.M. nodded again.

Dutton was feeling in fine shape. It looked like things were calming down and he'd weathered the VMAS fiasco now that the streets were almost back to normal. There would probably be more deaths here and there. These things never cleared up as you expected, but he thought he was out of the woods.

"You know I had to clean up that Ethan Taylor business. Can't have rogue reporters stirring up a big mess." Dutton took another sip of his drink, pulled the olive out of the glass and chewed it slowly. "Can we?"

"Whatever you think, Emory."

Dutton could see there was more M.M. wanted to say. He thought he knew what it was, but he waited.

When M.M. did speak his voice was desperate. "I need it now!"

"I see."

"The doctors say there's only a small window of opportunity left." Tears were welling in his faded blue eyes. "If I don't get it in the next week ... it's all over." He reached over and grabbed Dutton's hand. "Do you understand?"

"Do I look obtuse to you?"

"No, no, I would never say that, Emory. You know I wouldn't."

Dutton snatched his hand away. "Stop groveling! No more after this, you hear? Even the head honcho of News-Corp, who rarely lifts a finger, has to keep his wits about him."

"You're right, you're right. Absolutely. I promise. I'm finished with the booze."

But Emory Dutton knew they'd probably be having this same conversation a year from now ... if not sooner.

Dutton was beginning to relax. M.M., was obviously going to do what he was told. Without his constant cooperation and the pressure he put on News-Div, Dutton would have been in real trouble with the Corporit International Council. He didn't need to get into another cat fight with them.

I'm sick to death of the CIC and their interfering with how I run my business. They have way too much power.

Well, like it or not, sooner or later all those illustrious politicians would sit across from him begging for help. It was only a matter of time before everyone came face to face with their mortality.

That's when they all toe the line.

He looked at M.M. across the table. Maybe it was time to let him off the hook. He'd done what Dutton asked. Give the man the liver he needs to stay alive.

Especially now that he finally acknowledged who was really in charge.

Chapter 15

CORPORIT INTERNATIONAL COUNCIL
Emergency Committee Meeting

Adam Fiss, the Chief Supreme Interrogator, tapped his finger on the table where the other four CIC elected members sat next to him. Having that exalted position was like having a steel rod rammed up his back; it automatically made him sit up taller. After all, every country across the globe had agreed to adhere to the CIC's decisions. His decisions.

But it all had begun to get old and boring lately and he couldn't afford to entertain that kind of thinking. He knew this coming election was not going to be a run of the mill shoe-in. Not if the rumors were true. Not if that underground Defy organization was growing stronger.

What a bunch of fools.

The Corporits should have totally eliminated elections when they took control of the global governments. That's what Fiss had and still wanted.

Didn't have the balls. Wanted the people to have the illusion that they had control. Idiots!

He looked at the other seated members. None of them were actual lawyers. It wasn't until they were appointed that they studied any law. He was the only real lawyer at the table. But degree or not, they still represented global law—their decisions were final and there was no higher court to judge or reprieve given, unless this court changed its minds.

That had never happened.

Fiss remembered when he looked forward to these sessions—it would puff him up being the ultimate power force on the planet. It was amazing. The five of them could actually decide the life or death of a single individual, or shut down a mult-billion corporation. Their word was the final word ... throughout the world.

Now that was real power.

He looked at Argaret Charles, then at Cedra Cresting, better known as C.C. Both were tough but fair; Argaret was compassionate and easily swayed, but they were both excellent jurists.

Gary Blick was a downright fool and Marinda Bacha was a narcissist, just like everyone in that prominent family.

Fiss looked at his watch and banged a gavel. The meeting began.

"Mr. Slex, please stand. You are here representing Pharmcorp. Is that correct?"

The lawyer stood. "Yes, sir."

"Your client has requested this hearing concerning the misuse of the stabilizing patch by the Medical Programmers in the Sanfrancorp tri-state district. It that true, Mr. Slex?"

"Yes, it is, Chief."

"Please state your case." There was a brief pause. "Remember, this is a preliminary investigation. The court will only open these hearings to the public if this committee votes to do so. If not, your case will be remanded to the lower courts for arbitration.

"I understand." Slex pressed some buttons on his docuslate to read his notes. "Emory Dutton, CEO of the Sanfrancorp Medi-Progs, has violated a contractual agreement with Pharmcorp, causing us to lose a minimum of three billion dollars across the globe." He hesitated as he looked at his notes. "That's only an estimate. When the final figures are put into play, the loss could be much greater."

"And what is the agreement between the Medi-Progs and Pharmcorp, Mr. Slex?"

"It is quite simple, sir. All medical products, including vaccines, shall be produced and distributed by our corporation."

The chief bent over and conferred with four others. He finally said, "This *is* about the ineffective stabilizer that has taken the life of one million people?"

"Yes, Chief. The Medi-Progs had the tainted stabilizer compounded through a rogue pharmacy that also assumed the distribution."

The chief leaned over the conference table. "Now why would the Medi-Progs do that? They would have to bear the sole responsibility for that fiasco of all those deaths, when they could have rested it on Pharmcorp's financially stable shoulders, Mr. Slex."

"We are not concerned with the number of deaths. That is a collateral issue."

The Chief leaned back into his seat. "So you're not here because you are afraid of being blamed for the loss of life?" He snickered. "After all, that wouldn't have been necessary. Neither Pharmcorp nor the Medi-Progs would have been legally liable, not with the terrorists killing most of those victims. The Chief turned and spoke to the other members. "Luckily, terrorists fall under the clause concerning Acts of God."

Slex never took his gaze away from the chief. "It is sad that these people died prematurely when they could have had an existing, effective stabilizer that is under a low production level by our company. But, Chief, the death of those people are not Pharmcorp's issue. It's not why we are lodging this complaint."

"I see where you're going, Mr. Slex. You want your three billion dollars back, and you want it from the Sanfrancorp Medi-Progs for allowing another company to produce the defective stabilizer. In other words, the Medi-Progs violated your contract with them."

Slex let out a deep breath. "That is correct, sir."

The chief took only a moment to confer with the others.

"Okay, Mr. Slex. We don't think it will be necessary to go any further with this. You can now try to pursue your claim with the lower courts. Draw up your evidence for a full hearing down the road." He grunted under his breath. "And good luck with that."

"Sir, Pharmcorp had hoped for an ultimatum for payment from the Medi-Progs now."

The chief narrowed his eyes. "Slex, Advocatcorp has a good man in you, but you made the wrong call here today. You came here for money for breaking a contract. You might get it, but you're going to have to fight for it. You made it plain that the deaths of those victims were *not* your issue. Maybe the outcome would have been different if that was your suit."

"But, sir—"

"We are adjourned."

* * *

Dutton picked up the telelink right away when he saw it was Adam Fiss calling.

"Caught you before you stepped out for your two-hour lunch." Fiss laughed into the telelink. "You CEOs are really something."

Emory Dutton was uneasy and waited for the Chief Interrogator of the CIC to speak.

"We were in session this morning." The chief let it hang there for a moment. "It was a short meeting."

Dutton's heart was doing flip-flops as he waited. "And?"

"Oh, man, I'm just playing with you," the chief said, laughing. "It worked out for you, and they made it easy for me by presenting the wrong case. Not to say you and I couldn't have worked it out either way, as we have in the past." He hesitated. "Slex is a good attorney. I'm surprised he opened the wrong door to get this settled."

"The wrong door?"

"Let's just say, you might have to face this farther down the road, but ... let's see ... you only have a little over a year left and then you're out. Am I right?"

"Thanks for reminding me," Dutton said, feeling uneasy, as he did whenever anyone talked about him reaching mandatory retirement at age sixty.

"I doubt *you'll* have to face this in court. Pharmcorp may even drop it altogether. Those lawyers really charge a bundle and by then this'll be oooold news."

"Thanks, Chief. I owe you for this."

The chief let out a hearty laugh.

"Yes, you do. And don't think when the time comes I'll forget that."

Bette Golden Lamb

Chapter 16

CAPLAC DOMES

Zoe and Storm lay wrapped in each other's arms. She was dazed, her mind still spinning with visions of stars and brilliant flashes of color.

And it seemed they'd kissed a million times.

It was hard to trust again, but she'd surrendered to Storm, jumped into the void. Instead of it being empty, it was filled with love.

His hands ran down her spine, leaving behind bolts of pleasure.

"Zoe Hidalga, I love you." His eyes glowed, amber pools of peace.

"I love you, too." She wanted to stay right here, never leave. But that wasn't going to happen. "Storm ... you know I have to go."

He held her at arm's length. "I know you *want* to go."

"I'm alive, Laya's alive." She looked up to the sky beyond the dome. "Because of my friends, Nathan and Seka. I can't ignore that."

"Your friends wouldn't want you to risk your life in their name." Storm spoke softly, but she could tell there was an underlying controlled intensity. He ran his fingers through her hair.

"We can't let the Corporits continue to murder people. We can't let them win."

"This isn't a game, Zoe. Win. Lose. Those words have no real meaning. We win when we save people, save our earth. Lose if we don't."

"Maybe," she said, wanting to believe him, to never leave. She looked at his dark hair, then down to his strong chest. "Life and death are not just words. When you're dying, as I was only a short time ago ... well, my world and my perception of what's important have changed."

"You can do so much right here. You're a doctor with skills that can save people's lives. Can't you see that? Healing here is just as important as healing the Aughts or returning to Sanfrancorp where there's a death warrant waiting for you."

She leaned over to kiss him. "I can't move forward without settling the past."

Storm drew himself up into a sitting position. The passion he'd shown was now hidden as he morphed into a wise counselor. "All is chosen, Zoe ... you must choose your own path to enlightenment." He reached out, stroked her arm. "If you must continue with revenge in your heart before you can surrender to the golden path of enlightenment, then that is what you must do."

"If anything happens to me ... you will care for Laya?"

"I will always love Laya as my own."

* * *

Wolf was at her side as she wandered through the Aught territories. Two of Storm's closest companions also accompanied her. An amber eye rode the heavens after spinning out from a cloud of dust. Wolf's ears pointed ahead toward the land they would have to cover.

The men never seemed to tire and it looked like their feet barely touched the ground moving forward, searching for any danger.

"I have to stop," she said to one of the men. "I'm exhausted."

Wolf led the way to a niche in a scatter of rocks. She lay down in the partially protected spot, closed her eyes and drifted into sleep.

Intruders surrounded her, but it wasn't until Wolf growled that she became alarmed.

Storm's men closed in and the wolf shielded her with its body. It was early dawn. She could see the outlines of men almost upon her.

"That wolf belongs to him," someone said. She could see them looking up at the sky—the amber eye gazed back.

"Please! I've come to help. Your people are sick ... one of them has died at the domes."

The Aughts looked at the wolf and stepped away and Zoe followed them into the central encampment.

She stared at Godan, hated him. The man had once captured and tried to kill both her and Andrew Potter. But now he looked pathetic when he tried to stand and his legs collapsed under him.

"Get out of here," he screamed. "We don't want your filthy hands touching us. Your medicine made us sick."

She looked at the children covered in sores, ulcers that were infected. Dead bodies were scattered everywhere, each enclosed in a carpet of purple lesions. The rank stink of death wafted around them like an unholy presence.

Wolf hovered very close to her, snarling whenever anyone with a weapon closed in on Zoe.

She pointed to the fires surrounding their territory. "We have to dispose of the bodies." No sooner had the words left her lips than the dead were tossed into the huge bonfires by Storm's men. The Aughts began to help without being asked.

Everyone who could stand started cleaning the encampment.

Godan lay on his side and watched, too weak to do anything but glare while his people cleared out piles of human waste that had accumulated everywhere. All of it went into the fire.

There were three barrels of murky water. Zoe had the people use one of the barrels to wash themselves. Gathering the torn pieces of clothing that were lying in piles, she lined up the five remaining young children in front of her and stripped off their filthy rags. She washed them and tended to their wounds, had them put on some of the tattered clothes that were still better than the ones Zoe had burned.

She walked up to Godan. "Why won't you go to the domes? No one should have to live this way. You could have shelter; help to grow food and other plants to regenerate the earth. You could have a real life."

"This is a real life. What do you know about living free?" He spit on the ground. "You think I don't remember you, you bitch?" He raised a fist to her. "You and that black man escaped because the eye helped you." He pointed to two of his closest followers. "Get her and we'll do her as she should have been done before."

Two men circled in closer. Wolf growled and the wind started twirling around them; they looked at Godan and shook their heads, then stepped away from Zoe.

"Get away from my people. Get away from us. These are my tribal lands. This was my father's land, and now it's mine. Go before I kill you, you bitch!"

Wolf pushed against Zoe until she moved on.

Chapter 17

SANFRANCORP
Short Snack Restaurant

Jin Bacha couldn't believe it. The famous robotics surgeon and inventor, Andrew Potter, had called and asked her to lunch. He wanted to discuss a new neural synaptic device that could save many lives. The story would be for immediate news runs to the medical CEOs and he'd actually chosen her to release the story.

After the initial flush of importance, her usual doubts moved in to taunt her.

Why me?

Her Eurasian grandmother's voice echoed in her head, along with her old-fashioned homilies and spurts of ancient Buddha wisdom It alternately amused and annoyed her that even though Jin was twenty-six, her grandmother still called her a child.

Just accept your good fortune, child. Try not to over think everything.

But she knew why she'd been given this assignment. The CAPOs had taken Ethan Taylor away. He hadn't been around for a few days, so News-Div probably dropped her name for the interview.

Reality: It was probably going to be routine, boring stuff, not really big-time breaking news. Maybe someone else should have snapped up this assignment, but she wasn't about to let it go— even if the rest of the news staff managed to treat her like a dolt.

Where in the hell is Ethan?

That workaholic never missed work. He lived and died for any news story. Pushy as hell, but she liked the guy. They'd gone to lunch together many times and they'd always argued about political issues.

Ethan hated the corporations, always talked about how they sucked the juice out of the planet and didn't give a rat's ass about anything except making money.

Jin was unconvinced by many of his arguments, but his passion about the political picture always made her think, and feel uneasy. Still, Ethan was a down-to-earth man and his dedication to his work was inspiring.

Besides, she'd never heard of anyone in News-Div standing up to Medi-Prog CEO Emory Dutton except Ethan.

Everyone said the CEO was one mean critter and Jin believed it. At the last news conference, when Dutton looked at her—it was only a nanosecond before his eyes flickered away—she knew she'd stared into the iciest eyes she'd ever seen.

Just thinking about it made a shiver race down her spine.

It was one of those rare times Jin was pleased that she was nothing special to look at. She'd heard how Dutton snapped up beautiful women for sexual favors. That was the kind of corruption Ethan talked about. Jin hated it, too. And there were ugly rumors that those women were murdered when he was through with them.

Probably nothing but wild speculation. Still, Jin had tucked the information away in the back of her head.

That moment when Ethan stood up to the CEO made her proud to be a journalist. But she knew his getting thrown out of a news conference was the reason the head honcho of News-Div was still barking at all of the reporters.

Forget about Ethan. The CAPOs just took him away to scare the hell out of him. He was probably out chasing some woman's ass.

Let it go.

Over-thinking anything was usually what got her into all kinds of trouble.

* * *

Jin glanced around the upscale Short Snack Restaurant. It was fairly crowded, but there was no doubt everyone seemed to know Dr. Potter. He'd made a reservation so she was shown immediately to a table. Jin thought the Short Snack Restaurant was a misnomer. It was very elegant and after being seated, she took in the crisp, fresh tablecloth, and the bright red repli-rose in a graceful ceramic vase placed at her setting.

All around her entrees were being served to mostly well-heeled businesspeople. But when she looked at the walls, it annoyed her, as it always did, that all the decorative hangings were evenly spaced paintings that had no originality and displayed no special talent. It was the kind of bland corporit art that Jin referred to as industrial slush.

At least there was no one in corporit scrubs in this place. She was lucky that News-Div personnel were exempt from the dress code dictated for all other businesses. Today, she had on a beige dress with a chocolate brown suede belt that cinched in her waist, making her appear even more trim.

Guess they think forcing the dress code on reporters would ruffle the feathers of the press.

It was kind of humorous. Anything the Corporits wanted publicly blasted was passed onto News-Corp and sent to the News-Div networks—the Corporits had the press right in their back pockets.

That bothered her. She'd become a journalist because even though journalists were hamstrung, they still had the best opportunity to break out and let everyone know what was going on. She'd seen it happen. Ethan had done it plenty of times.

All she wanted was to bring news to the world. Real news. Instead, she was told what to write and most of it was obvious propaganda to terrorize the population into accepting the militarized CAPOs—she hated that murderous arm of the Corporits.

Now I'm thinking like Ethan.

Or maybe it was the Quinn legacy that made her question every single action by every single person. Maybe her cousin had really become a rebel.

The thought of him stopped her cold. She still couldn't buy the idea that he was a terrorist ready to bomb Sanfrancorp. That's what the Corporits claimed. But she knew Nathan. He'd always been such a gentle person, always tried to go with the flow. If he became a rebel, something really major had pushed his buttons.

But a terrorist? I don't think so.

Jin had gone to visit her Uncle Tris and Aunt Becky after she'd heard of her cousin's death. They were so sad and she'd felt helpless watching the two of them break down and cry, hugging, squeezing her between them.

Jin's husband Melik had totally bought the news story that told how Nathan and a cohort had tried to bomb the Corporit National Council headquarters, and how they were finally cornered in the Organ Harvesters complex. Melik claimed Nathan had become a tool for the underground Defy rebel group.

Jin and Melik had had a big-time blowout over it. Remembering it made Jin's stomach clench and her heart race all over again.

* * *

"I suppose the Quinns are above spying or bombing? They would never question Corporit government authority?" Melik had said sarcastically. "My little blossom, everyone can become corrupted."

She hated it when he called her that, knew they were in for a fight—something that had escalated in both numbers and intensity in the last year.

"You met my cousin Nathan," she shot back at him. "Did he seem like that kind of man?"

Melik smiled in the most irritating way, as though he had some special inside information that she could never understand with her tiny brain.

When he acted that way, all she thought about was how really stupid she was:

One night her friends had talked her into going to a local bar. She'd gotten wildly drunk and ended up in bed with a stranger—Melik. Remembering that night only made her hate herself. Jin had tried to convince herself it was real love. But the truth? She'd become trapped in a marriage with a horrible man. A man who would kill her before he would agree to a divorce.

"Still waters run deep, my sweet. And he was a man. That woman who went down with him was supposed to be gorgeous."

Jin exploded. "Don't judge every man by yourself—he wasn't anything like you, sniffing after every woman that crossed his path. Besides, you just hate it that my family is so well known and influential."

"I don't hate it. I just don't think they're that special."

"They *are* special." Jin pushed him away when he tried to take her into his arms. "Everyone, from my parents to Uncle Tris and Aunt Becky, has always worked in the medical field taking care of sick people." She put her hands on her hips. "And what have you done? Or your parents?"

"We're a filthy rich family that makes medical instruments, which allows us plenty of options. It's good enough for me."

"We've been married for five fucking years, Melik, and you're still wasting your time trying to impress me with the fact you're rich." She knew her face was getting red and splotchy. "So what!"

He looked at her with hate in his eyes for several long moments before he stomped out.

It had been a couple of days since that exchange and they still weren't back to "normal."

Chapter 18

Andrew Potter was jumpy. It was a huge risk to meet with Jin Bacha solely on his instinct to trust a Quinn. He'd looked into her background, trying to sniff out any kind of rebellion in her history that would at least make him feel better about what he was going to do.

There was nothing. To top it off, she was married to a Bacha.

Jin Bacha was past the age of just striking out at anything that crossed her path. She had a normal school record and snapshots of her gave him no clue as to who she really was. Her college scores revealed she was an extraordinary woman, grades at the top of the class. But even though her picture displayed an ordinary-looking person, there was an intense curiosity in her eyes—a penetrating search for answers.

Andrew had already spotted the tail following him, and knew he was now constantly being watched by Dutton's people. Changing the office staff was just the beginning and he knew the only thing saving him from instant disaster was his notoriety and respect as a scientist.

That bastard Dutton would love to plant me in one of the Organ Harvesters tanks—would do it in a heartbeat if he thought he could get away with it.

Still, if Dutton was set on doing him in, he would find a way. Andrew knew he'd better not forget that.

Maybe he would have to take up Storm's offer to move to the Noncorps area in the not too distant future. His days as a Corporit were probably drawing to a close, especially if he couldn't finalize the actions of the Defys and win an election during a short window of opportunity. The smart thing would be to walk away now. It would be easy and safe.

Safe as anything these days.

But the fact that the Corporits had murdered his parents because they dared to speak out against the dehumanization they saw all around them ... well, he couldn't let that go, couldn't just walk away.

* * *

Potter liked the Short Snack Restaurant; he actually came here often for a get-away long lunch. You could spend twenty minutes or two hours eating and talking without anyone trying to get you to move on. It would be interesting to see how the CAPO following him would be treated—he was dressed in clothes way too sloppy for the Corporits who frequented this place.

Then he saw Jin. She matched her picture in the News-Div employee news file, They had seated her in the middle of the room.

Perfect.

Andrew approached the table; a server hurried to his side. "Good afternoon, Dr. Potter."

Andrew ignored the greeting even though he recognized the man from previous visits. This is unacceptable," he said nodding at the table. All this in a loud voice and before he could be seated.

"Sir?"

Jin Bacha looked up. He could see she was puzzled. Andrew ignored her and frowned at the waiter.

"I specifically asked for quiet spot," he said in his nastiest voice.

Another server rushed to the table, looked around, pointed to a table against the wall. "Would that be acceptable, sir?"

Andrew took a long moment before he answered. "Yes, it would. Why wasn't it done in the first place?" Andrew held out a hand to Jin. She took hold and stood. The two of them followed the server to the new location.

"Yes, this is much, much better. Please bring us one of your best white wines."

"Yes, sir."

While they were changing tables, Andrew could see that the CAPO stalker was refused entry. Andrew couldn't help but smile.

* * *

Jin had eyed Dr. Potter walking into the restaurant. She'd seen pictures of the distinguished black scientist in their office files. The Internet picture didn't even begin to capture his formidable intelligence or his fiery eyes as he bawled out the server.

What the hell is he up to? Nothing wrong with this spot.

She had been enjoying a real lunch break without some News-Div executive breathing down her neck—she resented having to gather up her purse and move. But something strange happened when she grasped Dr. Andrew Potter's hand—he'd set off an electrical shock that still coursed throughout her body. It seemed a moment of surprise flashed across his face, even though it passed in an instant.

Jin sat down at the new table and tried to speak with an authoritative voice.

"Dr. Potter." Her voice broke and creaked. She was mortified. But he didn't seem to notice.

"Andrew."

"What?"

"Please call me Andrew."

The waiter held a bottle of Dobb's Chamaneau for the robotics doctor to view. He nodded, the waiter opened the bottle and poured some for him to taste. Jin could see the server was nervous after the earlier scene.

"That's quite good," Andrew said. The waiter's shoulders lost their tension. He filled their glasses and stepped away.

Bette Golden Lamb

Jin took a sip and warmth spread throughout her chest. The two of them had somehow left the restaurant behind and were caught up in a private world of their own. There was something magnetic, so timeless about the moment as they stared into each other's eyes. They continued to take small sips of the wine.

Finally, she said, "You have a new device we can talk about, Andrew?"

He hesitated. "I do ... but I don't know how to say this without seeming like a complete idiot. There's something going on between us ... something that I haven't felt for a long time."

His words made Jin's breath freeze. What was the matter with her? She was married. She should be offended. Yet, she sensed a primal connection to this man. One that she'd never had with anyone else.

"I don't believe in the kind of thing you're talking about," she said. "I ... I ... don't know what to say."

The waiter interrupted. "May I take your luncheon orders now?"

Jin had only glanced at the menu, but she ordered a chicken and radish salad.

"I'll have the same," Andrew said without looking at the menu.

* * *

Andrew was confused. This wasn't anything he'd prepared for. He was here strictly to try to plant Jin Bacha as a mole in the News-Div section of MediaCorp. The pictures of her hadn't hinted at the kind of sudden connection he felt for this woman.

He'd been divorced for several years but it was only recently that he'd truly severed an emotional connection to his ex wife. The last thing he needed at this juncture was a woman to distract him.

The waiter set their food down on the table, but neither took a bite.

"You're Nathan Quinn's cousin?"

Puzzlement clouded her face. "Yes."

90

"I didn't know your cousin very well, but during the short time that I did, he became a friend that I could trust and believe in." Andrew picked up a folk and shoved his food from one part of the plate to another before taking a small forkful. "Do you think he was a terrorist?"

She, too, played with her food and also took a tiny bite. "Do *you* think he was a terrorist?" She minced her words as though she couldn't swallow.

"I know he wasn't." Andrew reached across the table and took her hand. "He was a patriot."

Her breath was loud as she released it. "Why are they calling him a traitor?" Tears spilled down her cheeks. "He was my cousin and my best friend. I loved him."

"We only have so much time here." His shoulder hurt when he bent down and retied his shoelaces. As he sat back up, he did an eye sweep of the room. He'd only moved from the other table in case they had planted a bug when his reservation revealed his luncheon destination. Everything seemed okay.

She looked bewildered.

He pulled out a simplified schematic of a robotic device that had yet to be produced. One that would enhance robotic surgical skill. "Take this. You can use it to create a news release. But I must speak to you privately very soon."

"About what?"

"I will send you a request for clearance of your article before it goes live. Just to verify its accuracy." He took her hand again. "Will you meet me then? I'll explain more. Will you do that for me?"

She looked long and hard into his eyes. It was a moment before she smiled.

"I will."

Chapter 19

Jin went right back to work after her lunch with Andrew. Her time spent with him, from the first moment she saw him to the very end of the luncheon, had been confusing.

She tried to shrug off her attraction to the robotics genius, but it was hard to ignore her racing heart or the electrical thrill of his touch during that brief moment when they shook hands.

In the last year she and Melik had been fighting about every little thing. Any time she stepped away from the Corporit culture's standard answers to climate deterioration, medicine, and the collapse of services for the population, he would get furious.

"You talk about those people having rights. You know as well as I do that they have no privileges—those you have to pay for."

"People need help."

"Well, I think you like your privileges. I don't see you wanting to give up our fancy apartment." He gave a wave of a hand to take in the large apartment's living room, filled with expensive designer furniture. "Why haven't you walked away from Sanfrancorp or left to live with the Noncorps?"

"If I thought that would help in any way, I'd do it."

They would argue back and forth and it always ended the same way—he would stomp out of the apartment and Jin would immediately wonder if he was seeing another woman. He always came back after a couple of hours, smelling like he'd been rubbed in perfumed bath oil.

Jin sat at her desk and wrote a few news releases; mostly about the latest batch of terrorists who had left thousands of fellow citizens in the street to die.

The rumors were that the VMAS patch was what had killed everyone who wore them, but still the official word was the terrorists were to blame. There was no getting around it. Most of her work was writing about fear. Fear of the Aughts and rogue Noncorps.

The world changed in 2020 when the corporations seized control, took over and eliminated governments around the world.

It was no secret that Corporits only allowed continued voting rights as a means of silencing the rabble-rousers.

But over the years, protesters' voices seemed to grow softer and softer. Now that elections were around the corner and the Corporit political announcements were hot and heavy, Jin sensed a different kind of fear.

She remembered her Uncle Tris talking about what the electorate was like when they had some semblance of voice.

That was before the Corporit National Council handled all local disputes and problems and ultimate control rested in the hands of the five Supreme Corporit International Council members. Corporit rule across the globe remained in their iron fist.

Still, Jin knew, if the political leanings of the CIC board members ever changed, things could be quite different.

That seemed almost impossible. Every journalist in her office was sure the electronic votes were tampered with to favor hard line incumbent Corporit candidates.

She probably knew more about what was really going on than most people because Melik's sister, Marinda Bacha, was a sitting board member of the CIC. Jin already knew what her sister-in-law thought about everything.

She pulled out the diagram of the device that Andrew Potter planned to introduce when he performed his next surgery—the first time it would be used.

She studied the lines and realized there was something wrong with the illustration. When she pulled out a magnifying glass she could see interconnected in the center of the picture the words:

Join the Defys. We need you.

* * *

"Nothing I ever do satisfies that bastard," George Potek yelled at the walls of his apartment.

He'd been fuming ever since he received a warning from the CEO of his Corporit Aims Protective Organization that Dutton was threatening to pull the Medi-Prog account from their books.

And why?

Dutton claimed Potek had let the terrorists, Nathan Quinn and Seka Joraine, attempt to bomb the CIC offices.

What bullshit!

Potek had been right at Dutton's side when they'd vaporized the two "terrorists." They were in the Organ Harvesters complex when Dr. Hidalga and her daughter escaped. The two "terrorists" had never been near the CIC building.

All this because of Dutton's obsessive hatred of the Quinns. The CEO was determined to nail their asses no matter what he had to do, even if he used Potek as a football.

No! There was more to it. Dutton was covering his tracks for the massive deaths around the city from the stabilizer patch.

Maybe I am an idiot. I should have seen this coming.

Well, Potek was finished licking Dutton's ass.

This time he wasn't putting his tail between his legs and asking Dutton what he could do to make things better. This time he would suck it up and start looking for other options.

The commander eyed his small unit. Looking at this place you'd never suspect the kind of power he had over other people's lives. The power of life and death for anyone who crossed his path. He plopped down into his worn-out sofa. He lived like a drone.

A sharp pain stabbed through his middle , His stomach had been acting up and the doctors have warned him time and time again that his ulcers would do him in one day if he couldn't bring his crazy life under control.

Underneath all his anger, the thing that fired it more than anything, was his loneliness. He'd almost married twice. What always seemed to sour it was his twenty-four-hour commitment to Dutton. He couldn't remember the last time he'd gone a week getting a good sleep every night.

Now that his thirtieth birthday was coming up, he saw his chances of ever finding someone to share his life slipping away.

Potek knew all of Dutton's secrets. If the citizens of Sanfrancorp ever learned the real reason for the Organ Harvesters complex, they would string up Dutton and the CEOs. Most thought human organs were harvested and saved for their benefit, Little did they know it was a handy place for CEOs to get rid of their enemies or those who challenged them. Beyond that, with the constant replacement of worn-out or diseased parts, the elite Corporits could strive for immortality.

I'd better remember that or I'll end up floating in a tank, too.

Chapter 20

Zoe was at the very edge of Sanfrancorp's border, waiting at the station for a transpod. She buried her shaking hands in her pocket, then fidgeted with her blouse to cover up her rapid breathing.

For the moment, she had everything she needed to at least pass through the city. More or less up-to-date clothing—not the latest, but good enough. And there was her knowledge of the electric transpod system and how to transverse the city. But most important, she knew how the Corporits thought and the moves they would make to catch her. That critical knowledge might be the only thing to save her neck.

Still, she couldn't fool herself. If anyone took a real interest in her, they would become suspicious of her dated clothing, And, worst of all, her face could be scrolling across the telelinks people carried—it would not only show her picture, but create some horrible scenario of things she hadn't really done.

When the electro-magno pod pulled into the station, the door snapped open with a loud clang and she jumped back. A few of the waiting passengers eyed her, but she rushed inside and sat down in one of the single seats, trying to look uninterested by staring at the space in front of her, like everyone else usually did.

She was frightened and realized all her brave talk to Storm was false bravado that had nothing to do with reality. Everything she'd said to him was a front to hide how terrified she really was.

She'd prepared a plastin pack to protect her two piece corpiform of green and yellow that she'd raided from Arina Marek's closet. The clothes represented an obscure corporation that might not even exist anymore. In the past Arina must have come undercover many times to the city.

A man kept looking at her and she wondered if her picture had been on any of the building newscasts. Finally, she realized, her ID, which was an old useless one, was tucked into the folds of her blouse. She bent over to retrieve her purse, which allowed her ident card to end up on the outside of her top. It was too far away for him to actually read, and after a while he finally seemed to lose interest.

As they got closer to the center of town, more and more people filled the pod. The same newstrip flashed on and off across the ceiling:

TERRORISTS KILL THOUSANDS...ONLY CORPORIT RULE PROTECTS OUR CITIZENS.

Several men and women in the crowded car started looking her way. Her clothes must be giving her away, or maybe it was because she was scared to death, but she was catching their attention. She tried to breathe slowly, but her heart was racing, thrumming in her ears.

At the next stop, she left the pod at the last minute before the doors snapped shut. When she looked back through the window, two people had their telelinks pulled out and were engaging. She'd been spotted.

Zoe climbed the steps out of the station and hurried down the street. As she approached a corner, the CAPOs' sirens blasted and two vans pulled up to the station. The CAPOs filed out, looking like aliens with their black helmets hiding their faces. One turned and spotted her. He broke into a run, others followed on his heels.

She ran around the corner, sprinted down the street, turned another corner and mingled with a waiting crowd outside of a mall that was just opening. She elbowed, shoved her way to the front of the line and rushed inside.

She heard one of the CAPOS shout: "I saw her. She's in there. Seal the place off!"

Inside, people started screaming, scattering in every direction.

She looked for a staircase—there had to be one, it was a three-story building. Zoe's breath exploded in ragged bursts.

Have to get out now!

She pushed through an unmarked door and ran down a corridor that opened onto a loading dock—three trucks were pulled up to a ramp with their rear doors wide open. A hunched, older man stood at the back of one of them.

Zoe looked at him and froze.

His eyes widened. "Is someone chasing you?"

She frantically nodded.

He pointed to the interior of the truck. "Get in! Squeeze under the bottom of the cart in the back!"

Inside, she'd just pushed herself underneath a huge supply cart of shoes when she heard the CAPOs, their voices harsh and demanding. "Did you see a woman run through here?"

"What, am I supposed to do your job *and* mine. I don't see you helping me unload this truck."

The CAPO said something and the man yelled, "Okay, okay! Get your fucking hands off of me."

Zoe's heart was thumping, and she had to cover her mouth to help silence her breathing. She practically swam in the sweat, dripping from every pore of her body.

"Okay, okay," the man said. "Some woman came running out and took off down that alley. Now get lost and let a man do his work."

The truck shook as someone jumped inside. Loud noises blasted as a CAPO banged the different carts.

She stared at a pair of polished boots standing next to her hiding place. His feet kicked dust in her face and she held her breath, afraid of sneezing, afraid of swallowing.

"She's not here. Let's move on!"

It seemed like forever before the man reached underneath and pulled her out. "Easy now. I know it was a long time to be stuffed under there, but I wanted to be sure they were gone." He bent over and looked at her. "Are you all right?"

"I will be, thanks to you."

"I hate those bastards. They ran my sister over—she was just getting her little girl out of the street. The little one was just at the age where they love to run away from their parents. I watched those son-of-bitches mow them both down. Not even the beep of a horn to warn them."

Zoe started shaking all over. He looked closely at her. "When was the last time you had something to eat or drink?"

Zoe shook her head. "I don't remember."

"Well now, you stay in the truck—you can't go out looking like that anyway. You're kind of a mess. I'll go and pick up some clothes and bring you some food. Then we'll get you on your way."

Zoe reached out and hugged the man. "Thank you."

He was awkward when he patted her back—he pulled away, smiled at her. "It's all right. You're gonna be fine."

* * *

Becky Quinn was exhausted. She and Tris had been taking care of emergency cases for the last three days. Many of the doctors refused to treat people, to give any help at all, declaring many of the wounded were terrorists.

"A bunch of cowards. And they dare to call themselves doctors," Becky said, looking at her husband. "I think it's been so long since they actually touched a patient, they're probably scared to death they'll bite."

"The headlines continue to flash across the news strips and the internet. Over and over, they're saying, people are dead because of terrorists." Tris's face had blanched.

"That's what they called our Nathan."

"I know."

"A terrorist? They're saying our son murdered those people." Tris punched in the code to open the door of their apartment. "It's Dutton. How could he do something like that? Give them an altered patch. Set them up like that. What a horrible way to die."

"He's always warned that the number of people left on the planet would be critical for survival," Becky said. "Thousands died from the patch on their arms. The rest died from panic—trampled, beaten, knifed."

She stopped in her tracks. Tris came to a halt beside her. Both gasped.

Zoe Hidalga stood up from the sofa to greet them.

"Please forgive me for just barging into your home but I couldn't think of any other place to go that would be safe."

"Zoe?" Becky almost didn't recognize the woman. She looked wasted, but there was fire in her eyes. Becky could hardly believe it. The last time she'd seen Zoe was when she was a teenager. Becky smiled, then rushed to her, squeezed her close. "How on earth did you get in?"

"Nathan gave me the code to your apartment in case I ever needed it. I couldn't go to the old safe house—the CAPOs know about it."

Tris stepped up, took her arm. "It's been years since we've seen you ... you were just a kid."

"Without you, and your help in getting the real stabilizer, I would have been dead." Zoe smiled. "I know I still look like hell, but I'm getting stronger every day."

"Wait a minute, you were with the Noncorps and Storm. What made you come back?" He shook his head. "Dangerous." He moved to a chair and collapsed into it. "You should have stayed where you were, Zoe. You were much safer out of this mess."

"Nathan could have played it safe and maybe he'd still be alive, but he didn't."

Tris and Becky looked at each other.

"I have to do something," Zoe said. "I can't turn my back, leave it alone. I have to fight back. If it wasn't for Nathan ... and you, I would not be here today. You took a terrible risk for me."

Becky sat down on the sofa, patted the place next to her. Zoe joined her.

"Do you know how I can get in touch with Andrew Potter? I know Emory Dutton must be keeping a close eye on him. I don't dare try to directly get in touch with him."

"Why?" Tris said.

"I want to join the Defys. I have to help," Zoe said.

Becky took Zoe's hand. "You have your daughter again. Go back to where it's safe for the two of you."

"It isn't only about me. Sometimes you have to give up safety for something greater than yourself. I'm going to try to do that." Zoe said. "I want my daughter to be proud of me. I want to be proud of myself."

* * *

"They almost got me this morning," Zoe said, clutching the robe Becky gave her to wear after insisting she take a soak in a warm tub. The bath did help her to calm down. It was the first one she'd had in years since baths had been eliminated as a wasteful misuse of water. Of course, everyone knew the privileged probably had them. They were lucky. A hot bath was pretty wonderful.

"What happened?" Becky asked.

Zoe retold the story from the time she entered the city limits until she broke into the Quinns' apartment.

"You're a brave woman," Tris said.

"I was pretty frightened but there was no turning back."

"What do you plan on doing?" Tris moved into the kitchen and soon brought Zoe and Becky cups of tea.

"It seemed crystal clear when I was with Storm in the domes. But as soon as I breached the border everything I planned seemed frivolous and stupid."

"Tell us," Becky said. "Maybe we can help you figure out your next move."

"I can't involve the two of you. It's much too dangerous."

"And I suppose it's going to be a piece of cake for you," Tris said.

"We want to do something, too. We have to do something to bring Emory Dutton down," Becky said. "I know you understand."

Zoe looked at Nathan's parents—grief was etched in every line of their faces. She knew losing their only son had to be the biggest blow they'd ever have to live with.

"I don't know anything about the way the Corporit's inner circles manage the corporations, but I do understand every detail of the Organ Harvest division of the Medi-Progs." Zoe smiled at the couple. "If we brought that system down, I think it would have a definite domino effect on the Corporits."

"I'm not sure I understand," Tris said.

Zoe could see Becky was just as puzzled. Her face was filled with questions.

"Dutton has absolute control over who gets any of the organs in that facility," Zoe said. "Absolute control."

"Nathan told us about some of this and I know I sound dense." Becky shifted in her seat. "But, so what?"

"I've seen the files on the various CEOs who have gotten virtually new bodies from Emory Dutton's manipulations. You don't think he does that for nothing, do you?"

"Well—"

"Look, if you're going to die because you need a liver transplant, all Dutton has to do is tell you what he expects of you or there's no transplant. Those are the kinds of life or death sentences he can hand out." Zoe looked first at Becky, then at Tris. "The man is practically a king."

"Wait, what about the CIC? He can't have every member in his pocket."

"Don't bet on it," Zoe said.

* * *

What the hell does he want now? Potek thought.

He'd been summoned to Dutton's home and the two of them were sitting in Dutton's home office. The room had beautiful wood bookcases and a huge oak desk. Heavy carpeting covered the floor and made Potek want to take off his shoes and rub his feet in it.

My whole apartment is smaller than his home office.

"It's time I nailed the Quinns and you're going to help me do it, Potek."

The bastard treats me like shit and then he wants me to do his dirty work.

"Think of it as a big jigsaw puzzle." Dutton said, looking closely at Potek. "What's the matter, George?" You're not mad about that little ding I gave you with your company, are you?"

"The board is threatening to fire me."

Dutton smiled. "I just wanted them to nudge you a little bit."

"Sir, I don't need nudging to do my job," Potek said, not able to keep the resentment out of his voice.

"Look, I'll send a message in the morning, advising them how important you are to my operations. That ought to quiet their asses down." He looked intensely at Potek

Potek remained silent.

Scraps to a dog.

Chapter 21

Robotics Surgical Suite

Andrews's wounds were beginning to look as though they might actually heal. He was still on antibiotics but he could see that the infection had finally been beaten back.

Maybe all the extra decontamination he suffered for his Defy meetings was really an asset paying off. That and his Level IV Valek discipline. It had taken him years to master, but the technique of release and conquer had saved his life and sanity many a time. These wounds were no exception.

After the decontamination chamber, he walked naked into the surgical suite where everyone else, also naked, was waiting. No listening devices got into the meeting room when you're not wearing a stitch.

"B, C, D, am I always late, or are all of you exceptionally punctual?"

D said: "A little of both."

C spoke up: "I have to say I hate being called C. I understand the need for caution, but I just want to say I hate it."

He was always good for comic relief. They all laughed.

B: "I'm glad to see you're on the mend, A. Looks like you might actually survive that Aught attack."

D jumped in: "This is all very cozy, but we have elections in three weeks. Three weeks! My God! Let's get on with this."

B: "I'll just lay out the obvious. If we don't turn the CIC this time, we'll have to wait six more years."

C: "At least next year we're going to win in the regional Corporit National Council. We've finally got the CNC by the nuts."

A: "How did you manage that?"

C: "My eldest daughter and her lover, and her lover's lover are candidates for seats ... you know how they feel."

B: "But let's face it. The corporations have been in power since 2020 ... thirty years. They are not going to go softly into the night—"

A: "I think ... mind you, I think ... I may have found a way to push us ahead—"

"Wait a minute," B said, "did you say you might have found a way to push us ahead, A?"

Bang!

A crashing noise from the outer atrium shook the room.

All four of the doctors acted in unison—they folded themselves into gowns that they kept at the ready and immediately surrounded the Surgiclone, which simulated a torn carotid. They were supposed to be using a new technique to repair the vessel.

Commander Potek burst into the room using the emergency exit. Five of his CAPOs were with him.

"What's going on here, Commander?" Andrew Potter demanded. "This area is off limits —only physicians are allowed in the surgical theaters."

"A report was received that you are hiding a fugitive," Potek said. "We are permitted everywhere during a terrorist search."

B yelled at the commander, "Does this look like we're hiding anything or anyone, much less a terrorist?"

"We have to check it out," Potek said.

The marshals surrounded the doctors, ran their hands through the instruments and the tray to see if anything was somehow hidden in the metal pieces.

C laughed. "You checked it out. Now get your asses out of here!"

The commander glared at C, then looked at Andrew for a long moment before ordering the marshals to head for the exit.

Andrew yelled at Potek's retreating back, "Corporit Aims Protective is going to get a whopping bill for the decontamination and cleanup your breaking in here has caused. See how you like that!"

* * *

"Was she there?" Dutton asked Potek on his communicator.

"No, sir. She wasn't."

"Well, what did you find?" Dutton insisted.

"What I expected to find ... four doctors working on a surgiclone for practice."

"Did you search the whole room?"

"There's no place to hide in a surgical theatre. What you see is what you get." Potek let that sink in. "There was nothing to see, nothing to get, and no one hiding."

"Well someone fingered her in a transpod earlier today. She's in Sanfrancorp somewhere." Dutton hung up on Potek.

* * *

News-Div Offices

Jin Bacha looked again at the diagram Andrew Potter had given her at their luncheon two days ago. Their meeting had stunned and confused her. Was the attraction between the two of them only a ruse to get her into an underground rebellious group?

There was no one she could trust this with. She knew she was out of her depth and needed some advice.

Where the hell is Ethan? He's the one I always go to when things are muddied by politics. He has such a clear way of assessing problems.

She'd tried using the telelink to get in touch with him but there was no response.

Dammit, Ethan!

She'd not only called his apartment, she'd even tried to get his on-again, off-again girlfriend. She had no idea where he was either. The woman was pretty pissed though. They'd had tickets to a concert and he'd stood her up.

That didn't sound like Ethan.

Jin tried to do some nosing around, but just the mention of his name and everyone at News-Div clammed up.

There was no doubt in her mind now. Something really terrible had happened to her friend.

* * *

It was ten when Andrew's doorbell rang. He'd just come out of the shower. He wrapped a towel around his middle and went to the door.

Who the hell could it be at this time of night. If it's that damn Potek, I swear I'll break his neck.

He threw the door open, ready to scream his head off. Jin Bacha stood there looking up at him.

"I'm sorry to bother you so late, but..."

"No, no. Come in, Jin." He took her arm and led her to the sofa. "As you can see I wasn't expecting company."

"I'm worried about a friend of mine."

Andrew crossed his lips for silence.

"You know, I'm so glad you popped in. Let me get more presentable and we'll go for a walk."

She gave him a puzzled look, but said, "That's the best idea I've heard all day."

After he dressed, they left the apartment and were strolling down a well-lit street. He led her to a syn-park where they sat on a bench.

"What's going on?" she said.

"I think you know if anyone overheard our conversation, we might say something that could land you and me in real trouble." He reached for her hand. "Tell me!"

"My colleague Ethan Taylor is missing. I've tried everyplace, but he's vanished."

"Why do you think something's wrong?" Andrew said. Even in the dim light where he barely could see her, he felt his heart race. He couldn't help it, he was drawn to her.

"Ethan was thrown out of a press conference for standing up to Emory Dutton. CAPOs picked him up, took him away. No one has heard from him since."

"Are you fond of this guy?"

"Well, he's a friend."

"Let me look into it." Before Andrew could stop himself he leaned over and kissed her lips. "Forgive me. I don't know ..."

She reached over and drew his head back down to hers.

Chapter 22

Melik and Jin's Apartment

Jin woke with a start. She looked at the clock on the side table—it was four AM and Melik wasn't in bed. At first she sighed with relief. She could take the time to think more about what had happened between Andrew and herself.

They had kissed in that deserted syn-park, surrounded by all of those phony plants with their unmarred, shining green leaves on perfectly formed bushes that never came close to looking real.

* * *

Both were stunned by the explosion of passion that flowed between them. In the semi-darkness they kissed and kissed. Their hands moved over and under their clothes until they both pushed away from each other.

"What are we going to do about this?" Andrew asked.

"I don't know." It was all she could think to say.

"Why did you come to see me, Jin?"

She shook her head slowly back and forth.

"Tell me."

"I wanted to see you again ... but ... Ethan. I couldn't stop thinking about how the CAPOs took him away."

He held her head in both hands and looked deeply into her eyes. "I'll see what I can find out ... but I think you should be prepared for the worst. It's probably very serious ... maybe so serious there's nothing we can do for him."

"But I have to know."

* * *

She puffed up her pillow, tossed and turned and tried to push the memory of the two of them out of her head.

Finally, she stood, padded through the apartment barefooted. There were four bedrooms to look through—three were empty.

Melik wasn't in any of them.

She peeked into his office—she'd rarely been inside. He usually kept the door locked, but it was open tonight. A small desk lamp gave off a soft glow. He wasn't there, either.

She couldn't stop herself; she walked inside on the thick, dark-gray rug, ignoring the comfortable chairs and sculptures he had tastefully displayed. Instead, she moved towards his large mahogany desk and sat down. She felt like an intruder and she kept a sharp ear out hoping to hear him if he returned home.

She didn't dare get caught in here.

Jin looked at all of the odds and ends on top of the desk: a small picture of her, one of his parents. Many quartz rocks that were almost priceless; gold and silver pens—antiques that were rarely ever used.

Finally, she opened his desk drawers, one at a time. They didn't really contain much, not even anything relating to the work that he did for his father's company.

But there was a locked drawer.

She found a beautifully hand-carved knife at one end of the desk and she used it to wedge the drawer open.

The minute it slid open a picture of a beautiful woman stared up at Jin. She heard her own quick intake of breath.

A soft, "Oh" escaped her lips. This person was why he wasn't home tonight and so many other nights.

The woman looked about twenty. She had huge blue eyes and a luxuriant head of red, flowing hair. She was smiling at the camera in a soft, dreamy way. In the drawer next to the picture was a jewelry gift box. Jin flipped it open.

A large diamond ring was wedged inside. The stone caught the glow of the desk lamp. She gasped and immediately closed the box, put it back in the drawer. The drawer refused to latch again. She hoped he would think he forgot to lock it.

So Melik was having an affair. It didn't surprise her, but judging from the jewelry it was serious. She was shaken.

Does he plan on getting rid me, killing me?

Jin stood and put the chair back in exactly the same spot it had been, then gave the area one last intense scrutiny to see if there was anything she'd forgotten.

The knife was set back exactly as she found it, but her feet had left a map of indents into the rug. She bent down and backed out of the office, carefully smoothing away each step. When she finished, it looked as though no one had walked on the carpet since it was cleaned.

Out of the room, even half-naked, she wanted to run, run to Andrew, or just keep running. Instead, she went back to the master bedroom and tried to think of her situation rationally.

She was a reporter, but her influence was limited to being small and ineffectual. News-Div was definitely in the Bachas' pocket. There was no denying Melik's family was very powerful and her husband had a spiteful streak when he lashed out at others. Jin's father and mother were medical technicians and their connection to Uncle Tris and her Aunt Becky plus being a part of the Quinns were their avenue to power. It was like two different worlds.

She took a deep breath and crawled back into bed. She would pretend that she slept through the night and knew nothing of Melik's deception. She would feign ignorance until she could find a way out.

Chapter 23

Organ Harvesters

Andrew Potter stood at the entrance to the Organ Harvesters complex trying to work up the nerve to go inside. It was after midnight, not exactly the time anyone would be visiting the place, for any reason. But he'd agreed to help Jin.

He was confused about the woman. She also seemed confused about him. Was it strictly a physical attraction—if not, what did they want from each other?

He knew what he wanted.

He needed her to blast the city with the news that Sanfrancorp and every major city was in the middle of a Defy takeover—they would bring back governing power to the people. But they needed the news media to get the word out. It was unfortunate that he'd had to ask for Jin's help.

That had never been the plan—Ethan Taylor had been the Defys' first choice as a candidate for undercover work. But he was gone. And if he'd messed up with Dutton, he was probably permanently gone.

Yes, Andrew knew what he wanted, but what did she want from him?

He was a man of science, a cybernetic wizard. That's what the Corporits called him. What did he know about love? His marriage had failed miserably. People talked about love and destiny. Was there even a destiny, or a cosmic plan? Did he believe any of that was possible?

But Jin deserved to know the truth, especially since he would be asking her to risk her life.

He couldn't tell her what he thought really happened to her friend, Ethan Taylor. Not without proof. But Andrew knew the way Dutton operated. If Ethan was on Dutton's shit list, this would be the place to find him.

* * *

"That's right. I said between twenty-five and thirty years old—and he can't have been tanked over one week." Andrew made sure he was officious and rude to the night shift supervisor. Playing nice would get him nowhere.

"But why does it have to be a male?"

"Because that's what I want."

Andrew walked up to the computer she was looking at. Each individual had been turned into a number. There were fifty numbers listed. Ten were males. There were no names given.

"So, Ms. Lakin," he said after leaning over to read her name tag. "Where in this file are the names of the donors you have tanked?"

"Sir, that is privileged information."

"Yes, Ms. Lakin. And I am one of the privileged. I am the Chief of Robotics. You saw my ID when I was admitted to the unit."

The supervisor wore spotless white coveralls; she was wringing her hands. Before she could think any further about it Potter said, "Well, this isn't going to shine on your evaluation when I'm asked to give my opinion of your services."

She immediately tapped the screen and the list of names appeared, matched up with the tank numbers. It was like magic. There it was Ethan Taylor No54386.

"They all look promising." He indicated the reporter's listing. "Let's have a look at him."

She lifted the telelink and within a few minutes one of the staff appeared.

"Follow me, please."

"Thank you for your cooperation, Ms. Lakin. I'll be sure to note your compliance on your next evaluation."

Andrew followed the man down a corridor to a vaculift that took them up to the tenth floor.

"Step this way, please."

Andrew had been to this rotunda in the past. After seeing all the tanked human beings, he'd had nightmares for weeks afterwards.

He tried not to look in any individual tank, but he felt as if all the occupants within the watery holding tanks were following him with their fluid-filled eyes.

The escort stopped in front of tank No. 54386.

This was Ethan Taylor.

He was almost too big for the tank. Tubes pierced his rectum and abdomen—one vacuumed out body waste, the other was attached to the center's massive nutrient bladders that fed all the stored tanks. And there was a large tube that stretched Ethan's mouth open to force-fill his lungs with oxygen.

Andrew could barely breathe, but he asked with feigned indifference, "Have they ever reversed any of these specimens—released them?"

The escort looked at Andrew as though he'd fallen from the sky. "I cannot answer that question, sir."

"And why not?"

"Because I don't know the answer."

Andrew tried to look away but he forced himself to take a long, final look at Ethan. He was curled up and backed up to one side of the tank, as though he were trying to get away from someone.

His wide eyes blinked back at Andrew.

Bette Golden Lamb

Chapter 24

Caplac Domes

Asher Wind Storm looked at Tabo, the fierce leader of one of the last of the Aught's rebellious tribes. He had decided to save what was left of his people and request to live in the domes.

Many Aughts had come to Storm to join with the Noncorps to tend the Caplac Domes' farms. Tabo and Godan had been the last of the major tribes to remain on the outside.

Storm knew Tabo's people were now as decimated as Godan's. Both tribes had stolen medical supplies from the CARE units to save their sick members from a certain VMAS death. They died anyway.

"The Corp'its lied. Just as they always do," Tabo said to Storm. There was fire in his eyes and venom in his voice.

"You have to put that hatred behind you if you are to survive here in the domes."

Tabo sneered. "I will never forget what they did."

Storm eyed the rest of the Aught's tribe. If they left now, they were doomed. There were only six children. No babies. Storm knew these women would never have any more children. They were starved, tired, and wasted. They had the barest of flesh left on their bodies and it would take a long period of recovery before they were whole again—if ever. It was obvious that most of the available food had gone to feed the men. But even they were thin. Every single person in Tabo's tribe would soon die without food and rest.

Tabo understood this. It was the only reason they were here now.

"To stay with our community, Tabo, you will have to put destructive feelings of revenge behind you." Storm reached out and ran his fingers through Wolf's fur as he spoke.

The animal had refused to leave Storm's side since they'd entered the healing dome. This dome was filled with the most diversified of plant life—most came from the vestiges of the oldest rain forest. Storm often came here to meditate and breathe in the aromas of each plant. No other place enhanced Storm's healing powers as this one. It was here he'd also brought Zoe to gather her strength.

"Why do *you* help the Aughts?" Tabo couldn't stop looking around in wonder and even though he tried to hold onto his anger, Storm could already see changes in his personality—anger was slowly ebbing.

"Many of the Aughts' different tribes have already come here to work and live ... anyone can remain in the domes as long as they are willing to work the land. We need you as much as you need us."

"We're tired," Tabo said. "And there's very few of us left. We're too weak to work."

"You will heal, become strong again. But until you do, you can stay in this dome." Storm moved in closer to the Aught. Wolf stepped forward with him. "But like the other Aughts who have been welcomed into the community, you will eventually have to work with the land in these domes."

Tabo stared at Storm.

"I only repeat this because you have to understand the terms. Nothing changes that. It is the one absolute condition of acceptance. We grow all our own food, and remember, the Caplac Domes hold the future life of the planet. We all need each other to survive."

"We don't think about the future."

"You'll learn. And you'll be responsible for the dome you live in. Every plant, every seed will become your personal responsibility." Storm held out his hand. "That is the pact you must agree to. Otherwise you can leave now in peace."

Tabo turned to his people. Everyone nodded their agreement, even the children.

The leader took Storm's hand.

* * *

Storm traveled through many domes for the rest of the day. In each one he ran his fingers through the soil. One touch told him not only the condition of the dirt, but how healthy the plants inside were.

As his hands probed the layers of the earth, the filaments of his own substance would reach out to every living thing within.

Everything is connected. All is one.

When he was a child, his mother would take him from dome to dome. It was a ritual she performed until he was a grown man. She would always say the same thing: "Feel the golden threads of life ... feel them intertwine with yours ... let the magic of life move through you to them, and them to you. Know this is a bond that must never be broken. It is our connection to the land that allows us a place in the universe."

When he was eighteen, she no longer had to say the words, but he could still hear her voice in his head.

Every time.

Shortly after his eighteenth birthday she died. That was when he began to hear the voices of the wind, of the rain, of the earth, of the very air he breathed. And without warning, one day he morphed into an all-seeing eye that traveled through time and space. With these changes came tremendous powers, and although he was never sure how it had happened, he had become so powerful his abilities required extreme discipline to control.

It had humbled him as great power always should.

He closed his eyes and allowed the world to slip away. The air flowed through his hair and, with his arms held out like the wings of a bird, he flew through space and time until he was lifted up, up into the higher realms.

Tonight he narrowed his vision to see the city of Sanfrancorp below. He searched and searched for a special essence.

From the many beams of life, Zoe's shone like a beacon.

Chapter 25

Sanfrancorp

Zoe was still in a room the Quinns had given her to rest until they could reconnect with Andrew Potter. She was exhausted, yet she tossed and turned, moved from one end of the bed to the other.

It was in the middle of the night when she sensed a presence. Her eyes snapped open—she looked around, but there was only darkness and silence. Soon her lids grew heavy. She began to float ... float ...

A breeze flowed around her; soothing fingers ran over her body. She was on the same ledge she'd been to before—high above the earth. It was black everywhere except for the blue glow of the earth below her.

Beautiful. So beautiful.

She wasn't frightened at first, but when she looked down at her feet, there was only room for each foot on a feathery ledge— bit by bit, it was falling away into space.

Zoe heard Storm's voice. It was everywhere.

"Zoe, come back to me."

"Where are you, Storm?"

"I am everywhere."

"Where?"

"Everywhere."

Zoe stretched, reached out into the void.

Awoke with a jolt.

* * *

Sanfrancorp Apartment Complex

Andrew was deep in concentration. Deeper and deeper he dropped through the layers of his mind as he worked Valex's exercises of deep mind stimulation. He took a cleansing breath— his doorbell rang. The sound snapped him back to the present moment like the splash from a bucket of cold water.

"Damn! Who could that be this early?"

He flung the door open. Tris Quinn stood there looking wasted, as much in shock as the day Dutton murdered Nathan.

"Tris, come in. what are you doing here this early?"

"Just wanted to drop by." Tris reached into his pocket and pulled out a piece of paper.

"Have a seat. I'll make us some tea." Andrew took the paper with him into the kitchen.

The note said: *I know you're being watched. Need your help. Zoe Hidalga is at our apartment. Must get her to a safe house. She insists on seeing you.*

* * *

Safe House

Tris, Becky, and Zoe went to the address that Andrew had written on the same piece of paper Tris had given him. She could see how frightened they were but it didn't stop them from accompanying her.

They left at Zoe's insistence the minute she arrived at the unit. It was in a low rent area.

Strange, Zoe felt more at ease in this district than she did in the upscale streets where the Quinns lived. People were less likely to be interested in strangers here.

The last safe house Zoe had been in had elegant furnishings, exciting paintings covered the walls. This place was only a single room. A small bed was folded into the wall and there was a tiny area where she could make something to eat, plus a sink to wash up at. There was no shower.

124

She'd hardly been gone from the Noncorp zone but she missed the domes. The thought that her daughter was again separated from her made her uneasy, but at least Laya was with other children and Storm was watching out for her.

Thinking about her little girl made her smile with happiness.

It was midday before there was the sound of someone standing outside of the door. Zoe tensed, ready to fight or take flight if she had to. But it was Andrew. She ran into his arms. He hugged her, then held her at arm's length.

"You look like a different person. You're starting to get some color back in your cheeks. Dare I say, healthy looking?"

"Between Storm and the patch I'm healing, Andrew. It's all working."

"Then why in hell would you come back here with a death warrant hanging over you and Laya?"

"Laya, too?"

"You know as well as I do, the goal is less population." He sat in the only chair in the room. "That's what Dutton's Desisto Processing is all about. Did you think they would hesitate to kill a child? Both of your pictures are all over the telelinks."

"Laya is safe with Storm."

"And that's where you should be." Andrew smiled at her. "So why are you here complicating my life again?"

"I want to be a part of the Defys."

He quickly stood, started pacing out the small area. "I know how badly you want to hurt Dutton, but there's nothing for you to do—other than keep me on edge worrying about you."

"I may be new at this, but I can see what has to be done—start breaking down the choke-hold the Corporits have on the population."

He smiled at her. "I told Elliot he was selling you short, that you *could* be a part of the Defys."

"No, I think Elliott knew me all too well." Sadness clutched at her heart at the mention of her dead husband. "I just didn't understand or even care about what was going on. Truth be told, I was perfectly happy with my head buried in the sand."

"It's certainly easier than facing the realities we're all stuck with." Andrew returned to the chair, sat down, and looked up at her. "We have a very narrow window of time to get done what has to be done."

"I know."

"And you've chosen a crucial time to come back to Sanfrancorp." He was up and out of the seat. He paced back and forth in the small unit, finally stopping in front of her. "Redemption is near and we *will* take back what was stolen from us."

She reached out for his hand.

"And I think I know how I can help."

Chapter 26

Corporit Hospital

Becky Quinn had gathered eight of the most influential medical chiefs in a small, rarely used lab. Tris insisted she be the one to call the meeting because even though he still worked as a consultant, he no longer retained his voting power since officially retiring.

The eight doctors had passed on the necessary information by word of mouth. Everyone stayed off the internet, using no electronics to discuss the meeting. If Emory Dutton ever caught wind of it, they would not only be in deep trouble, they would all end up dead.

Tris knew many who would still be willing to stand up against medical Corporit control, but the numbers were growing smaller with each passing year—most doctors were afraid of being caught, being labeled terrorists, of being killed. Worse, it could mean they might end up entombed in one of the Organ Harvester's tanks. They all knew others who had already met that fate. Dutton had already managed to eliminate some of their most influential people.

Although the Defy movement was a secret global call to arms, Sanfrancorp was at the core of the entire rebellion because it was at the core of Emory Dutton's power base.

For many, especially the very youngest doctors, Corporit medicine was all they'd ever practiced. Soon there would be no one like the Quinns or the eight other physicians in this room, willing to stand up to CEOs like Dutton.

There had been six sanctioned CIC elections since the corporations took power and everyone suspected the votes had been fixed in favor of the Corporits—most found it hard to believe this coming election would be any different. The big question: Why had they ever allowed the people to vote in the first place?

During the early years of Corporit rule, they had been leery of deleting the elections —that it might stir up massive rebellion. But now there was talk among the Corporits and the CIC of eliminating elections altogether.

The Defy proponents within the population knew they must win the upcoming election or it might be all over.

The room was in the bowels of the Medi-Prog building. It had been neglected and it smelled musty. The eight doctors sat around a grime-covered conference table staring at each other. Tris knew how they felt—they'd rather be almost any other place.

"All of you know what Emory Dutton did to our son," Becky said, opening up the discussion.

The Chief of Communicable Diseases said, "It was horrible. Dutton has no honor."

Pediatrics spoke up. "Or conscience. He labels everyone who disagrees with him a terrorist ... and it works every time."

"It's a clever method," Tris said. "Keep the masses living in fear for their lives and they'll do anything for the illusion of safety."

"The planet's dying. For God's sake. There is no safety," the Chief of Oncology blurted.

The Pediatrics spokesperson took a quick sip of water from a glass sitting in front of her. "It all gets down to having the same corrupt people running the CNC and the CIC."

Hematology's chief said, "They have all the power ... we have none. What can we do?"

"We will withdraw our services," said the Radiology Chief. "That's our clout."

"Who will coordinate all of this?" The Chief of Communicable Diseases asked. "We all know our only hope is to replace the sitting members of the CIC by voting them out, and we have to shut down all of our services at the same time. How do we even accomplish that."

Another asked, "What about the CNC?"

"We think the Corporit National Council will fold in the same way when their elections are held next year." The soft-spoken Dr. Doran, Chief of Radiology, said, barely above a whisper. "But all of us have to declare ourselves, get behind the same candidates now."

Becky looked long and hard at the imposing doctor. "Declare ourselves?"

"I am a Defy member. This is not news to any of you. All of you will have to join the Defys, too. We must have one global agenda—focus on the vote. On election day, the world will shut down all medical services, including the CARE units It's the only way."

The Chief of Radiology said, "Are we all agreed?"

They all turned to Tris and Becky.

"To the elections." They both raised a fist.

* * *

George Potek had been alerted about an illegal doctors' meeting somewhere in the Medi-Prog facility. That was the only info he had.

He'd been sitting in his office after a long, unsatisfactory meeting with Dutton. One where the CEO had treated him like a fool, as usual.

On Potek's orders, his team had planted bugs in every room of the building. The area the group of doctors was spotted in had a very low priority, but one of his newest recruits had caught the activity and had called him immediately.

"Sir, it's probably a glitch but there is voice activation in a room in a basement lab."

"Corporal, thank you for reporting this. Nothing is to be said to anyone else." Potek paused for emphasis. "Is that perfectly clear?"

"Yes, sir. Of course, sir."

Potek tapped into the room in question. He listened to the recorded back-and-forth conversation and immediately understood the direction of the treasonous actions of the doctors.

Well, well. It looks like our Emory Dutton has a mutiny on his hands.

Potek sat back in his desk chair and smiled.

* * *

Emory Dutton was restless. His instincts told him Andrew Potter was up to something, yet none of his usual traps seemed to be working. Not even the changing of Potter's staff, putting the lovely Regina in as his assistant seemed to be producing any useful information.

The woman was beautiful, chemically enhanced with pheromones specially formulated for Potter's tastes—yet nothing had happened. It appeared that Potter was totally uninterested in her sexually.

Dutton studied the activity schedule and analysis of the robotics genius.

Potter had had lunch with Jin Bacha, but Potter had a new procedure he was touting and that wasn't such an unusual kind of meeting. Besides, that particular reporter from News-Div was married to Melik Bacha. His family was one of Dutton's most loyal backers.

They damn well better be, with all the medical instruments the Medi-Progs purchased from their company.

Jin's father-in-law, Roger Bacha was a member of the Corporit National Council. His daughter was a member of the CIC. Both did whatever Dutton told them to do.

If I remember correctly, Roger Bacha has a perfectly matched pair of kidneys and a new liver in that body of his. And it was all because of me.

Poor guy called me to the hospital in tears. Seems some kind of poison caused a massive cascade of toxicity in those vital organs. Hell, it might have been his own son, trying to get rid of him, according to Potek.

Without Dutton and his Organ Harvesters operation, Bacha would have been a spot on the wall.

But it sure did make him a loyal subject.

He thought about Potter again. There was that raid Potek carried out at the Robotics Surgical Unit. Dutton had really had his fingers crossed on nailing him in his own operating room.

Such poetic justice.

Nothing!

Maybe that Dr. Zoe Hidalga they spotted in Sanfrancorp was up to something that had nothing to do with Potter.

Maybe. Maybe. Maybe.

First they needed to find the woman.

Bette Golden Lamb

Chapter 27

Sanfrancorp Safe House

The noon hour was the best time to slip away from Dutton's stalkers. Andrew went to the nearest transpod station and pushed his way into the middle of the lunchtime crowd. Right now he was being followed by only one man—at least that he could see.

Why the hell do they always dress these guys in jock outfits?

This man probably could have been a jock if his body movements weren't those of a couch potato, and for some reason he kept sniffing at the air as though there was some secret scent to follow.

When the pod arrived, Andrew acted like he wasn't interested in its destination. But at the last minute he jumped into the pod as the door was closing. Through the window, Andrew could see the stalker grabbing his telelink to have someone else pick up the trail. He got off at the next station and grabbed a pod going in the opposite direction.

The safe house where he'd stashed Zoe was only a block from the station. With minimal exposure he was inside. As far as he could see, he was in the clear.

"Where have you been?" Zoe said the minute he walked through the door.

"Hey, you have all you need here. It's not like I don't have a job and other things to do."

"I'm sorry, Andrew. I've just been so antsy locked up like this."

"It's better than being dead, which is what you'll be if they ever catch you."

"I know." Zoe sat down on the bed, which she hadn't bothered to stack back into the wall.

Andrew sat down in the chair. "I don't know exactly how to tell you this, but I think I'm in love." He gave Zoe a wide smile and watched surprise cross her face.

"Hey, it's been a long time," Zoe said. "Anyone I know?"

"No. And she's married ... into the Bacha family."

Zoe sat up taller. "Isn't Roger Bacha one of the members of the CNC? And his daughter on the CIC?"

"Guilty, as charged."

"Man, you've got to be crazy, or you've got a huge death wish."

"I know," Andrew said, looking away. "It just happened ... believe me, it wasn't anything I was looking for. The last thing I need is someone other than you to complicate my life, especially someone whose family we're trying to unseat."

Zoe gave him a dry laugh. "Tell me about her."

"She works for News-Div ... she's a reporter."

"Uh-huh! You sure you're not mixing up someone you need help from with instant love?"

"I wondered that, too, but we just seemed to ignite around each other. It was spontaneous. I couldn't ignore it. I tried. She should be here any second."

"Andrew, are you crazy? She could expose you ... expose me."

Andrew shifted in his seat. He was a scientist and wasn't usually one to take a leap of faith about anything. He could just imagine what would happen if his Defy cell knew what he'd done—no, he knew. They'd make life a living hell for him. He shifted in his seat. His mind was racing. For all he knew she'd be here any minute with the CAPOs.

What an idiot I am.

* * *

Andrew and Zoe both stood at the door and listened to the tapping from the other side.

She knew there was no place to hide in this unit. Would this be the moment they would finally trap her. Andrew looked terrified as he grabbed the door knob and snapped it open.

A Eurasian woman stood there, looking up at Andrew. Her eyes were soft and dreamy. It was hard to tell her age but she appeared to be in her mid twenties. He grabbed onto her and pulled her inside—then they were in each other's arms.

If this wasn't love, then Zoe didn't know the meaning of the word. Holding onto each other they seemed to morph into one person.

The woman reluctantly stepped away and turned to look at Zoe. Her face reddened. She said, "Hi, I'm Jin. You must be Zoe, Andrew's friend."

When Zoe took her hand she could feel the woman trembling. "Sit down." She pointed to the bed.

"No, I only have a few minutes ... I have to get back to work." Jin turned to Andrew. "Were you able to find out what happened to Ethan?"

"This is going to be hard, Jin."

Her eyes widened and Zoe could see fear flash across her face. "Tell me," she said to him.

"It might be better if I didn't."

"Please. I have to know what happened to my friend." Her voice was trembling as she clutched his arm. "Is he dead?"

"No. But he might as well be." Andrew looked away.

"What do you mean?"

Just looking at Andrew, Zoe could tell exactly what had happened to Jin's friend. "Sit down," she said to Jin, leading her to the bed.

"Tell me!" Jin said again.

Andrew sat down next to her and took her hand in his. "They're ... they're ...

"Jin," Zoe said very softly. "They'll be taking the organs from his body for implants into others."

"But you said he was alive," Jin said, tears spilling down her cheeks.

"He is for the moment," Andrew said. "For his sake I hope it's not very long."

"Where?"

"At the Organ Harvesters complex," Zoe said.

"Let's go and get him. Now that we know where he is, we can bring him home."

"What they've done is basically murder him," Andrew said. "It's too late to get him." He took hold of Jin's arm. Zoe could see her skin being pinched from his pressure.

"Why have there been no stories about this? I thought that complex was for storing organs for people who need them." Jin kept swatting at the tears that refused to stop.

"They are being stored."

"I don't understand. If he's alive, how is that possible?"

Zoe and Andrew stared at each other.

"For God's sake!" Jin screamed. "What are they doing to him?" She looked at both of them. "Tell me."

"They've stored him in a tank ... tubed his stomach and lungs to keep him alive so they can use whatever they want from his body ... when they want it."

"Oh my God! No! Does he know ... is he aware of what's happening."

"I think he is," Andrew said. Zoe nodded at the same time.

Jin's face was a mask of frozen hatred. It took several long moments for her to speak. "You asked me to help bring down the Corporits?"

Andrew nodded.

"I'll do anything ... anything you want."

Chapter 28

SANFRANCORPS
Dutton's Office

The CEO of the Med-Progs was restless. Things weren't coming together the way he envisioned. His jigsaw puzzle—an analogy Dutton liked to use concerning his leadership—was scattered all over the place.

He had hoped to have another Quinn trapped and quartered by now, but again Tris and Becky Quinn had managed to outsmart him. Everyone was talking about what heroic figures they were, taking care of the sick and dying who besieged the hospitals looking for medical care.

Damn it! It's my own fault. That accelerator patch not only caused people to drop dead in the streets, it also created uncontrollable panic and trauma injuries.

Pretty sophomoric of him to think they would die at home in their own beds. He'd actually thought that was the way it would happen when he came up with the plan to accelerate VMAS. Now, because of his stupidity he had to continue to sell the populace on the unlikely notion that terrorists had attacked the city.

He didn't misstep often, but this was a big one. Most of the doctors were angry and mistrustful of him—not that they weren't already. But they were even more so now.

With elections coming up, his timing had been all wrong and if the members of the CIC were unseated, who knows what kind of sanctions would come his way.

Right now I have those illustrious rulers in my pocket, so I need them to win their elections, keep their seats.

Potek had assured him that he kept a huge dossier of misconduct on each existing member on the CNC and CIC. Enough to hold them all in line. And that wasn't even taking into consideration the organs that Dutton had been supplying those bastards to guarantee them a chance at immortality.

Yes, he had more than enough on those supercilious idiots who thought they could tell him what to do.

Good old Commander George Potek will probably save my ass again if he does his job. And why wouldn't he. He's nothing but a young punk who better do what I tell him—or else.

Dutton stood at the penthouse office window. The dome covering the city was close enough to view outside the amber covering—he could see the bay from this height. Just the right distance so he didn't have to actually look at the garbage-choked waters. He knew at the very edge of the dome lay the filthy sea and a whole colony of exiled Corporits living in houseboats.

Stupid idiots would rather die on the polluted bay, breathing the polluted air than go to the Noncorp city centers.

Thinking about it just made him more restless. For a moment he considered running home and sitting back with some music, something that would calm him down, but then he'd have to see his wife, Barbara, with her black straggly hair and stony eyes. She'd jump on him for coming home in the middle of the day and bothering her.

Just a vision of his wife was enough to agitate him. And the fact that she had outsmarted him was a constant flash point.

For years he'd been trying to figure out a way to get rid of Barbara, but she was always way ahead of him. She'd safely stashed everything she knew about him, and that was plenty, in a hidden place with instructions to Advocatecorp to make it all public if *anything* happened to her.

The mistakes we make when we're young keep haunting us.

Maybe a quick trip to his mistress, Taura, to indulge himself in an hour or so of intense sex would calm him down.

He picked up the telelink and put in a call to Clinton, his limo driver. He knew how lucky he was. CEOs were the only ones allowed a private limo and he used the privilege as often as he damn well pleased. Within a minute a call came in from Clinton's company.

"Hello, Mr. Dutton. How are you today?"

"Where's Clinton? I need him."

"I'm sorry, sir, Clinton has the afternoon off."

"Unacceptable!" Dutton said in a harsh retort.

"Sir, I can get Edgar to drive you anywhere you'd like."

"Fine! Get him here in five minutes."

"I'm sorry, sir. The streets are still clogged with cleanup crews. Is fifteen minutes acceptable?"

"No!" He yelled into the telelink. "I'll expect him here in no more than ten minutes. Is that understood?"

"Yes, sir. We'll try our best."

"Not good enough!" he screamed.

When he disconnected he picked up an engraved glass award—*CEO of the Year*—flung it across the room. What the hell did he care if it broke, which it did. He received a new one every year.

* * *

Dutton stood in front of the Medi-Prog building, pacing back and forth. He'd been waiting fifteen minutes when the chauffeur, in the long, black limo, pulled up to the curb.

The driver jumped out of the front seat, tipped his hat, and opened the passenger door for Dutton.

"Hello, sir, my name is Edgar. Sorry to be late, sir. I couldn't get here any sooner."

"I don't want to hear it," Dutton said, climbing in the back.

When the driver was settled, he said, "Where to?"

"The James Complex."

"Yes, sir."

He and Taura had a standard appointment once a week and he'd just seen her two days ago. It was an arrangement they'd

139

had since she became his mistress two years ago. He had other women—many of them—but they were seen in a different apartment he kept for disposable women.

Yes, that's how he thought of them. Women to fuck and palm off to the Organ Harvesters complex in Sanfrancorp. Many body parts from those fine specimens had been used, some even transferred around the globe to other Organ Harvesters satellites.

None of those women ever lasted more than one or two encounters. He didn't like complications in his life, so they became the disposable ones.

But Taura had turned into a not disposable woman.

Dutton wasn't sure how it had happened, but she had gotten under his skin. She fit every fantasy he'd ever had about the perfect woman and she never disappointed him

He reached into the hidden liquor compartment and poured two fingers of Alexandra Golden Brandy into a cut-crystal tumbler. He held it up to the light before downing it in one gulp. He'd only meant to take a small sip. Instead of soothing him, it agitated him.

What's the matter with me today? I can't seem to hold it together, no matter how hard I try.

But he knew what it was. In one month he would be fifty-nine years old. Leaving him only one year in his powerful position as CEO of the Medi-Progs. After that he would be nothing.

"Shit!"

"Can I help you, sir?" Edgar said over the intercom. "Is there something wrong?"

"Shut your mouth and drive." Dutton reached for the bottle of brandy, poured himself a generous refill, and then another.

* * *

The James Complex

When they arrived at The James Complex, Edgar quickly came around to Dutton's door and opened it.

"Shall I wait here for you, sir?"

As Dutton stepped out of the car his ankle turned, pushing him off-step. He fell into Edgar and couldn't help but notice the ripple of muscles on the driver's arms as he caught Dutton and kept him from falling face first onto the sidewalk.

"Are you all right, sir?"

"I'm fine. Yes, wait here for me. I'll probably be about an hour."

"Yes, sir."

Dutton tapped in the code, waited impatiently for the vaculift. When it arrived and he stepped inside, it took him to the twentieth floor in five seconds. He rarely used the code entry to the apartment and today was no exception. He held his finger on the buzzer and didn't let up. When there was no answer, he tapped in the door code and stepped inside.

Taura came out from the bedroom in a bra, naked from the waist down.

"Darling, what a surprise. Did we have an appointment to meet today?"

Dutton's eyes narrowed as he moved into the bedroom, took in the rumpled bed. "Appointment? I don't need a fucking appointment. You're mine! Remember?"

She moved closer and threw her arms around him. "Of course, I only meant I didn't expect you and I just went back to bed for a little nap."

He pushed her away and reached out, ripped off her bra and tossed it aside. She moved up against him, rubbed her breasts into his chest and whispered in his ear, "Take your clothes off and get comfortable, darling."

Dutton started to kiss her but the musky odor of sex enveloping the room was not only female. She'd had a man here.

"Who's the man you've been fucking?"

Her eyes widened, not in surprise, but terror. "Emory, darling. What do you mean? You know there's only you."

He threw her onto the bed and moved to the huge walk-in closet, flung open the double doors. Standing inside was his chauffeur, Clinton. Dutton eyed his naked body, starting from the top of his head and moving down to his toes.

"So this is what you do with your afternoon off."

"Sir! I'm sorry."

"You haven't a clue as to how sorry you're going to be."

Dutton pulled out his telelink from his jacket pocket and tapped in the number for George Potek.

"Get down to Taura's. There's some pickups for you."

Clinton grabbed his clothes, which were in a heap next to him on the floor of the closet, and tried to dress in a hurry.

"You can try to run, you miserable piece of shit, but I have other plans for you."

It seemed like only seconds had passed when the buzzer rang and a voice called out, "It's Potek. Open the door!"

Dutton took his time, walked to the door, and flung it open. Potek followed Dutton back to the bedroom.

Dutton pointed at Clinton. "Take him! You know where."

Potek grabbed Clinton by the arm and turned to Taura.

"Take her, too!" Dutton said.

"Emory, please. I didn't want to do it. He forced me."

Taura tried to grab for a blouse lying next to the bed. Dutton reached for it, threw it across the room, and nodded at the robe on the chair. She grabbed it and covered herself.

"It was him!" Her face was a mottled red. Drool was running down the sides of her chin.

Clinton yelled at her. "Liar!" He yelled out to Dutton. "She started it. It was her!"

"Potek, get them out of here. Now!"

The commander also latched onto Taura's arm and pulled the pair of them out of the bedroom. Dutton followed in their footsteps.

Clinton had not only become the disposable chauffeur, Taura had now become one of the disposable women.

Chapter 29

CORPORIT INTERNATIONAL COUNCIL SUITE

The Chief Supreme Interrogator eyed the four other CIC members who sat around the oval conference table. All of them looked as bored as he was.

Adam Fiss hated dinner meetings when he knew that everyone, including himself, would rather be home. Although he was rethinking that idea, too—when he was there, he was destined to listen to his wife moan and complain again and again about their teenager's activity as a building jumper.

What the hell was the matter with the younger generation that they needed to swing with steel ropes from building to building, amputating their arms or bashing their heads? And they call it a sport.

His son never bothered to listen to him anymore—he still did two or three swings per week—even after his best friend had turned into a vegetable from spilling his brains on the side of a building. The only reason the kid was still alive was because the top robotics neurologist had saved his life. Thinking about it gave Adam the shivers. That kid would have been better off dead.

Adam Fiss forced himself to look at the other four members of the board, all of whom were staring back at him, waiting for their special dinner orders to arrive.

He turned to Marinda Bacha. Damn, if she wasn't the ugliest woman he'd ever laid eyes on. It was a good thing she came from the wealthy Bacha family because she wasn't too bright, either.

Cedra Cresting kept clearing her throat as she always did when she was nervous. She was the rogue member of the board.

C.C. didn't always go along with what was thrown her way. She had a lot of newfangled ideas that people should have a say in the governing process. He'd been beating her back for five, going on six, years since she'd started getting so many rebellious ideas in her head. It was getting pretty tiresome.

Gary Blick's eyes were drooping. He always had trouble staying awake for their meetings—day or night. He and Marinda together still wouldn't equal one decent brain no matter how many cells they intermingled.

Argaret Charles was a real pain in the ass. Another do-gooder. It seemed to Adam she always voted against anything he voted for.

Trays of food were finally wheeled into the conference room by waiters in crisp, white jackets, wearing white gloves. All had raven hair with black eyes and jutting chins. Their voices even sounded alike. The three of them looked as though they'd been cloned from the same donor.

Everyone had opted for food from Asher Wind Storm's domes. No one wanted the ersatz vegetables and chicken from a cafeteria in Sanfrancorp, even though Adam doubted any of them had ever eaten in a cafeteria. He knew *he* hadn't.

"Dig in," Adam said. "I don't want to be here all night."

"Have any of you ever visited the Caplac Domes where Asher Wind Storm grows this food?" Argaret took a large forkful of peas and mushrooms, chewed slowly. "Because this is delicious."

"I have," Adam said. He pushed his vegetables to one side of his plate and cut into the chicken breast, covered with a tart, lemony sauce.

"What was it like?" Argaret asked.

"The first time I took a tour." Adam put his fork down and thought about the experience. "But after that, I've gone to visit them at least once every year—"

Marinda Bacha interrupted. "Why on earth would you want to visit that heathen's domes?"

"Ask me, the man's kind of humorous, running around in Indian gear," Gary said, laughing, his mouth opened enough to show the bread he was chewing. "Looks like he belongs in some of the old vids they called Westerns." He laughed again. "Did you ever see the ones with the scalping?"

C.C.'s fork clattered to her plate. "What on earth is the matter with you, Gary? Who would want to watch that disgusting act of barbarism." She leaned over the table and made no attempt to hide her contempt. "Sounds to me like you're the savage sitting at this table."

"Why do you want to make fun of the person who puts the food on the table?" Argaret's face had turned a bright red and she all but had steam coming out of her nose.

"That's enough, you two." Adam took another bite of his food and sipped his vegetable juice. "To answer your question, Marinda ... visiting the agricultural domes was an intoxicating experience."

"Intoxicating?" Argaret asked.

"The minute you walk into one of those structures, you're overwhelmed with aromas that are pungent and laced with the musk of wild plants floating in the air. I used to smell those odors when I was a child. They were everywhere. It's heady... and Storm has wildlife—domes with deer, rabbits ..."

"Oh, so what," Gary said. "I say get rid of him and his domes. All they do is take up space—"

"I swear, you don't have half a brain," Argaret interrupted. "In case you haven't noticed, this planet is dying. Our one glimmer of hope is something you want to get rid of? You're a fool, Gary!"

"That's enough," Adam said. "Let's get to the reason for this meeting and stop tearing each other apart."

"Good idea," Marinda said.

Adam dabbed at his mouth with his napkin, then threw it on the table. "We've got an election breathing down our necks.

If any of us are replaced ... well, things could change drastically."

"I don't know why we haven't eliminated these silly elections," Marinda said "It's just a formality anyway. Most of us have been in office for almost half the time since the Corporits took over in 2020. Things aren't going to change ... ever. Except that maybe we'll get rid of these stupid elections every six years."

Adam could feel himself getting fired up. He took a deep breath and said, "Sorry, Marinda ... that's a pretty naïve attitude. Underground Defys have been growing in membership. We don't know their exact number but I think they're enlisting more and more converts from all over the world. These are people who definitely don't like the way we're running things; They've turned into a secret political party." He shifted in his chair as a tingle of worry rode his spine. "The info we have is damn disturbing."

C.C. blurted, "I agree, Adam. They're definitely becoming a force to be reckoned with."

"Nothing but a bunch of stupid Noncorps," Marinda said.

"These are *not* Noncorp outcasts," Adam shouted. "The Defys are Corporits like you and me. And they're trying to bring down the Corporit system—bring it all down. They're right here among us and across the globe. With the elections coming up, it's the best opportunity they've had in six years. They could send us walking out the door. Gary, you could find yourself back in Oslo, me back to my hometown in Germany. I like living in Sanfrancorp."

Gary jumped to his feet. "This is all bullshit."

"Remember, including us, there are nine people running for the five Council seats," Adam said. "The challengers are Mitchell Payette, Olga Yammo, Hani Singer, Podes Diaz. Only one of them isn't worrisome."

"Who? Gary said.

"Mitchell Payette." Adam had gone to primary school with him and they were still pretty good friends. "His father is the CEO of Germany's Pharmcorp division."

Marinda and Gary both laughed out loud.

"Hell," Marinda said" Get with it, Adam. We're all going to be fine unless we die of old age sitting in these chairs at one of these endless and boring meetings."

Chapter 30

Emory Dutton's Office

Dutton listened carefully to Adam Fiss. The telelink became very heavy and a rush of discomfort made his feet tingle.

"I don't know, Emory. I'm beginning to really worry about the upcoming election. That challenging slate of candidates sounds solid. Not like the usual idiots they drag up to oppose us."

"You've always assured me that none of you would ever lose. That they never would have a decent challenger." Dutton shifted in his pneumatic chair, waited impatiently for it to readjust itself. "What's new to the equation?"

"Defys."

Dutton's chuckle sounded phony even to him. "Six years ago they hardly existed. Why the big change?"

"You really must live in an ivory tower. They've been growing in numbers. We know that. And no one really knows how many there are. It's not as though we can go from door to door and take a census."

"Very funny." Dutton wasn't smiling.

"As I said, this list of candidates is pretty solid." Adam sounded exasperated. "They're young, ambitious, and they've made no bones about the facts."

"Facts. What facts?"

"What facts?" Adam Fiss said. "You've got to be kidding."

Dutton was really getting fired up. "I've never been much of a kidder, Adam. So lay it on me."

"The deteriorating environment around the globe is killing more and more people with respiratory failure, cancer, heart failure, malnutrition. Shall I go on?"

"Hell, we need less people," Dutton said with a dry laugh.

"You keep on saying that, but when the air's gone ... when we can't breathe anymore ... it'll all be academic."

"That's it?" Dutton said. "That's the facts you want me to face."

"Don't you get it? We're running out of food for the masses," the Chief Supreme Interrogator said. "If it wasn't for Asher Wind Storm, you'd probably be eating dirt pancakes along with the rest of the population."

"What I'm hearing, Adam is a lot of whining."

"Call it whatever you want. When people start to vote, that's just some of what they'll be thinking about."

Dutton didn't like the growing unease nesting in his stomach. "Are there any of the new candidates that'll be in our corner?"

"Only one. Mitchell Payette." The line went silent for a moment before Adam spoke. "He's the only one."

"Let me think about this, Adam." He managed to blurt out a chuckle. "Don't worry ... you know I always land on my feet."

Adam didn't sound too confident when he said, "I hope you're right."

* * *

Emory Dutton stared up from his desk chair at George Potek. The CEO slowly bit off chucks of his morning Danish and washed it down with his special blend of corpcaf while the commander stood shifting from one foot to the other.

When Dutton finally had consumed the pastry, he said, "Tell me what you know about the Defys."

"There's really nothing to say, sir."

"And you don't think that's a problem, you fool?"

The commander lowered his eyes.

"My understanding is they are a growing segment of resistance in the population that could cause us real problems." Dutton suddenly banged his hand on the desk.

Potek flinched.

"And all you have to say is—'there's really nothing to say?'"

"They're a very secretive group divided globally into small, non-centralized cells, and that makes it difficult to nail any of these resisters." Potek's eyes met Dutton's. "We don't have enough information ... as yet."

"Well, if you don't want to end up out of a job or turn into some ass-licking marshal, I suggest you get over those difficulties."

"Yes, sir!"

* * *

George Potek couldn't remember the last time he was this angry. His heart was clawing its way out of his chest and he could barely catch his breath.

He jumped into the back of a waiting hovervan. The driver said, "Where to, sir."

"Take me to the nearest syn-park."

The driver shifted in his seat and stared at the commander.

"You heard me."

They drove on. It was more than a week since the VMAS riots and crews were still cleaning up the mess from the dead bodies that had clogged all the avenues in the city. Usually there were a few stray walkers ambling about, but today, with the exception of the cleanup people, the streets were almost deserted.

That's the last time he's going to treat me like a piece of shit.

The seeds of a plan were starting to grow within him.

Fire me? Lower my status? That bastard Dutton would probably finish me off one way or another without thinking twice about it. He can't afford not to. I know every move he makes, everything about his operation. He has no secrets from me. And that means he'll have to bring me down.

Potek remembered the last time he visited Organ Harvesters. It was the day they trapped the Quinns' son in the dissection-vaporizing unit. He thought about that day a lot lately. Nathan Quinn and his lover still lived in the corners of his brain.

"Is this syn-park all right? the driver asked, interrupting his reverie.

Potek sat there for a minute and looked out the window. The place looked rundown. Many of the phony plants had been pulled out of the ground and were lying in piles. Unlike real plants that were yanked out of the ground, they were still green with that waxy glow, but still they ended up looking like just ordinary trash that needed to be picked up and taken away.

Potek stepped out of the hovervan and walked to the park. There wasn't another soul in the area. His thoughts were confused. He'd always followed orders from the time he was a teenager. His mother had taught him that fighting the system was useless. Look what had happened to his dad.

Dad had helped erect the Organ Harvesters. In fact, he was one of the primary designers. When he discovered the real reason for the facility, he'd refused to work on the project any longer. Potek was in his teens when they came and dragged him away. That was the first time he'd seen Emory Dutton.

Potek had been standing on the sidewalk outside his apartment complex getting ready to go inside when his father was dragged outside and thrown into a van. Before they closed the door, his father looked into Potek's eyes—there was both rebellion and sadness.

Dutton had walked up to him and placed a hand on Potek's shoulder.

"Do you know that man?"

"He's my father."

The hand was quickly withdrawn.

Potek watched his mother. She had followed the marshals out of the building when they took his father out. She was screaming for them to leave him alone. At first she was angry. But she ended up begging them to let him go. Potek could still visualize them pushing her away like she was nothing.

He sat down on the syn-park bench. He hadn't thought about that day for a long time, but now everything that happened fifteen years ago was very clear in his head.

Bette Golden Lamb

Chapter 31

The Domes

Storm stared at Andrew Potter's message. The words tore at his heart:

Storm,

> *I think you're in love with Zoe or at the very least, I know you care about her deeply. Right now, you need to intervene, step in and take her away from the violence and terror that is about to explode in Sanfrancorp. The Defys are in the final stage of reclaiming our government. It's now or never. If we can't accomplish change in this next election, all will be lost for many, many years. It may never happen. The Corporits have to go down, or not only will human civilization disappear, the planet will be completely uninhabitable. And sooner, I fear, than any of us really know. Taking away Corporit power could be bloody, very bloody, and I don't want anything to happen to Zoe. I made a promise to keep her safe. I know she respects you and I also think she's in love with you, so I need you to step in and help me with this. She simply won't listen to me.*

Andrew

When Storm read the robotics doctor's note he had to quash the overwhelming urge to find Zoe and steal her away from Sanfrancorp.

He could not.

All life was his mission.

157

His powers were a gift, given to him to help heal the dying planet. That was his sole focus from the time he was a very young child.

Nothing had changed.

Saving all life still remained his primary mission.

No matter whom he loved, there was the greater love for the land that had been placed in his protection. First, by the souls and ancestors of his people. Then by an unspoken universal force.

There were no answers. Only questions. Why had his destiny been altered, stolen away from a normal path of life? He did not know.

He only knew that all life had to be saved.

From the beginning, he'd struggled with his human part, the part that wanted to live in peace and quiet and love. But a universal calling had been permanently etched into his soul. It would override everything and everyone.

The domes were his mission. All life would remain his mission.

* * *

Storm sat in the center of his closest followers. They had been chanting and meditating for many hours. He would know when the moment was right. Then, he could rise with the winds that circled the sacred hill.

A pipe was passed among them. They smoked a healing substance that grew in Storm's special greenhouse in one of the largest domes. He'd been with his mother when she uncovered this sacred plant in the very last existing rainforest. It grew nowhere else on the planet.

Many of his followers had tried to nurture the seedlings, but only Storm's hands made it thrive.

He rose. A vision of Zoe appeared before him. He moved towards her, but the universe opened up to him and he left her behind.

Rising, rising, a gust of wind enfolded him in its cushioning billows.

He rose, rose higher, and the earth below fell farther and farther away.

Soon he was among the stars that shone with a brilliance he had never seen.

Bette Golden Lamb

Chapter 32

SANFRANCORP
Andrew Potter's Apartment Complex

Andrew was deep into sleep when callused hands grabbed his arms and yanked him out of bed.

"What the—" A hand clamped down over his mouth.

"Not one more word or so help me I'll taser you until you turn into nothing but a blob of jelly. Do you understand?"

Andrew nodded.

Something was thrown over his head and he was dragged to a chair. Rough hands yanked on his clothes and shoes—then he was pushed along, staggering, into the elevator. After that, he was tossed into a vehicle.

His heart raced with terror. From inside the pitch black hood, the only things he recognized were a stink of sweat and the low murmur of voices he couldn't quite understand.

The vehicle bumped along for what seemed like about twenty minutes before it came to a stop and they threw him out of the vehicle. Their footsteps echoed as they dragged him into a building that made him think of a musty warehouse.

"Put him in that chair. And tie him down."

Andrew's rump hit a steel-hard seat. His arms were yanked, yanked so hard behind his back he thought his shoulders would pop out of their sockets.

"Do you need us any more, Melik?"

Andrew heard the solid smack of a fist connecting with a jaw.

"Owww! God dammit, why'd you have to do that?"

"I said no names. What about that is so difficult to get? Even someone as dumb as you should understand that."

Andrew knew they had to be in a fairly large space considering how far away the voice was resonating.

Melik? Oh, shit! This must be Melik Bacha, Jin's husband.

"Do you know whom you're talking to, big-shot robot man?"

"I haven't got the foggiest idea. What the hell do you want with me?"

Andrew grunted as he was back-handed across the mouth.

"I'm the one asking the fucking questions here. Are we on the same page now?"

Even with the cloth over his face Andrew's cheek was stinging. He nodded, listened carefully, but now he was almost positive that there was no one else left in the room except him and his lover's husband.

Is that a good thing or a bad thing?

He tried tugging at his bound hands. They were tied tightly and there was no way he was going to get loose. At least for now.

"I really haven't decided yet what the hell to do with you." Melik coughed and then there was a series of heavy hacking. Finally, Melik's throat cleared.

Jin's husband probably had severe allergies and with good reason. Even Andrew could taste the heavy dust under the thick hood. Melik started pacing around him. Andrew sensed the tension surrounding him.

"I'm here to ask you some questions ... I won't lie to you. If I don't like the answers, you're probably going to die right here ... tonight. Do you understand?"

"I understand."

"Do you know Jin Bacha?"

Andrew could feel a trickle of sweat riding down his back. "Sure, she's a reporter for News-Div."

"Are you having an affair with her?"

"What?" Andrew burst into a roll of laughter. "Are you kidding me?"

"I assure you, doctor, this is no joke."

"No! I barely know the woman."

"Do you always go to lunch with women you don't know?"

"This is ridiculous. I went to lunch to discuss a new surgical procedure that I will be introducing in the near future. That's all."

Andrew felt a tug at his bound hands and the rope was suddenly loosened. Then there was nothing but silence.

"Did you hear me?"

Silence.

"Hello," Andrew called out.

"Son-of-a-bitch!"

It took Andrew at least an hour to work his hands free. When he finally pulled loose and could yank the hood off his head, he saw his hands covered in blood from grinding his wrists against the fiber.

As he suspected, he was in a huge empty space. He'd been set in the middle of what was obviously part of a vacant warehouse. It wouldn't be difficult to nail down who did this, or who owned this place, but why go through it all when he already knew Melik Bacha was behind the whole mess.

Her husband must keep close tabs on Jin.

I better remember that. And so had Jin.

Bette Golden Lamb

Chapter 33

Organ Harvester Complex

It was midnight when Zoe left the safe house, scared, but determined. The two blocks to the transpod station seemed like miles, but the streets were deserted and so was the station as she went to the tail end of the platform.

Her movement activated a large hologram of a pointing finger. It warned whoever saw it to vote for the existing CIC members or terrorists would end up at your doorstep and kill you.

> These are the people who will take care of you. Bring them back!

Holographic names hung in the air as it presented the lineup:

> Adam Fiss
> Cedra Cristing
> Marinda Bacha
> Gary Blick
> Argaret Charles

Within a few minutes a second one popped up—it had images of all the actual candidates lined up. They stood and smiled and reached out a hand.

Zoe had heard about the pop-ups in the stations from Andrew. He'd said Cedra Cristing and Argaret Charles were not thought to be part of the Defys, but they were independents looking for change. He felt they might do the right thing.

She stood against the wall and thought about the candidates as she waited for the pod.

Bacha? Wasn't that Jin's sister-in-law?

What has Andrew gotten himself into?

She knew about the Bacha family. They were the corporation that made the special instruments for dissection at the harvesting labs. Zoe, of course, had used them.

The transpod arrived, pulled up to the platform. No one debarked from the line of pods. They looked empty. In fact, she'd seen no one since she left the safe house.

It was good luck but it was also creepy—like traveling through a dead city. She stepped into the pod and chose a corner seat, hunched down to make herself smaller, but she couldn't stop trembling as she waited for the final stop on this line—The Organ Harvesters Complex.

She left the station, tried to walk in the shadows of the pathway in case there were patrols skirting the area.

It was very quiet.

Memories crowded her head with every step. Zoe thought of the Quinns and their generosity to her, how welcoming they were when she was a teenager in love with Nathan.

The last time she was here was the night that Nathan and Seka died. When she and Laya had escaped from Sanfrancorp. Thinking of them made her sad, but it also gave her the courage to go on.

She passed the park and turned to look at the large Nicola Fountain—its metallic petals used to glisten with the water bubbling over, sliding across the shining metal. It was one of the few remaining fountains that still had circulating water cascading over the huge sculpture. Most of the others in Sanfrancorp were now kept bone dry because of the drought that had been with them for decades. This fountain was the only perk that existed for the people who worked in the Organ Harvesters. She used to eat her lunch in the park that surrounded the sculpture. It always felt like a moment of freedom.

Zoe looked up at the sky and felt secure for a moment knowing that Storm was out there and would be waiting for her to return.

Storm. Her daughter, Laya.

* * *

Zoe had Becky Quinn's ident-card around her neck, but would it be enough? She remembered how Nathan's mother wouldn't take no for an answer when Zoe tried to give the identification card back to her.

"Zoe, please. You have to use it. I hate that you're even going back there, but if you must go, my card might be just enough to get you inside that nightmare facility."

"But even if I get inside, they'll have a log-in using your name. Dutton hates you and Tris."

"Yes, he hates the Quinns and always has. From the very beginning we've been able to gather enough medical clout to stop some of his worst ambitions."

Becky Quinn had looked away and Zoe knew she was thinking of her lost son and how all of this might be just what Dutton finally needed to destroy their reputation once and for all.

Zoe heard the sound of an approaching vehicle, then saw the lights of a patrol unit checking the park. She fled to a side entrance and slid the ident-card into the machine.

The heavy metal door snapped open and she hurried inside. A chill coursed through her as it clanged shut behind her.

At least this complex didn't require finger ID. Who would want to come into this place if they didn't have to? Most people had never seen the complex—it was the last stop on the transpod and most of the population only knew of it as a medical storage house for organs if *they* needed a transplant.

167

Ignorance really is bliss. Like the average Corporit was ever going to get a single organ from this depository to save their life.

Zoe stood still and listened to the sounds all around her. Memories flooded the moment, memories of how she'd spent each working day of her life here in a laboratory where she had to dissect one human organ after another.

Her job was easy compared to the doctors who had to dissect the living subjects in the tanks. Most of those doctors only lasted a year, if that long. They went mad, usually killed themselves or ended up in the tanks, too.

A chill jolted down her spine. All she wanted to do was run.

She took deep breaths to fight the panic. Stood her ground.

Zoe had asked for this—she was the one who begged Andrew to let her help in any way she could. At first, he'd refused, but there were answers he needed and time was short. It would have to be a person who knew the facility well, knew what to look for. Only a hands-on approach would work. If it meant coming back to this miserable place, Zoe was ready to do it.

The whole complex had turned into a private world of its own. Not only self sustaining, it had its own energy production units and all of its systems were separated from the Sanfrancorp central communications and control centers.

Emory Dutton had isolated everything.

The roaring in her head finally settled and she could hear the voices of the guards talking to each other. Andrew's informants had revealed there was only supposed to be a minimum of protective personnel at this hour, but whether it was one or one hundred of them, they were all a threat.

Most of what she heard were the familiar sounds of working machinery, the constant hum of pumps providing oxygen to the tank occupants. There was also a strange, continuous click-click-click-click that resounded throughout the complex. She'd not heard it before and she couldn't identify it.

Zoe edged into the main rotunda, tried not to look at the huge tanks spread across the bottom layer of the area, but she couldn't help it. People were trapped in solutions, with tubes piercing their bodies—it was impossible to look away. She stared above, studied three nutrient bladders, realized there used to be only one. But the numbers of live people had grown and they must have needed more providers to feed all of the specimens. That was how these trapped people were referred to—specimens.

Zoe thought about the solutions. Where were they prepared and how did they fill the feeders?

She kept down low as she headed for the staircase. The emergency exit door was ahead—she took the ident-card and slid it through the information slot. She held her breath until the door lock released. Any irregularity would set off an alarm.

The door remained open for barely enough time for her to slip through, but there was no alarm. When it returned and latched, she ran for the staircase and moved quickly up the steps to the seventh level. She used her card again and the door slid to the side.

This was the floor where her laboratory was when she'd been part of the system. She ran, circling the floor until she came to central control. She knew exactly where it was because she and the other doctors were warned to stay away. They usually had a guard outside the door, but at this hour no one was there.

She tried her ident-card again, but the door wouldn't open. Instead the mechanism guarding security requested an eye-scan. It would be the end if she tried that—she knew there was a kill-on-sight order for her.

She was not getting inside the room. There was an opening to view the chamber but it was only a slit. Zoe stood on tiptoes and peered inside.

The first thing she saw was a huge glasstron vat with finger controls for making solutions.

She could see where they mixed the nutrients for the people in the tanks and could barely make out the label on the machine: ***Genetic Variation Solutions***

Without this everyone in those tanks would die.

Next she saw what was probably a techtron station for the robotic unit to output the neural sequence technology. In the far corner of the room, there was a spot she could barely visualize. The energy panel was housed there. This had to be what kept all the internal systems for the tanks working.

Andrew was right. No one outside of the Organ Harvesters could tamper with the tank system, or anything in the whole complex. That's why Andrew didn't have the necessary info. Everything that kept the subjects and the organs alive was generated from this one room.

Zoe straightened. People were walking down the corridor, laughing. They would turn onto the arc that would expose her in exactly one minute.

Chapter 34

Zoe's ears were thrumming. She bit down on her lip and held back a scream, took off in the opposite direction, back to the emergency exit.

No, No. It would take too long to open. Their voices were getting closer and closer. In a moment they would grab her.

She raced around another corner, rushed to the dissection laboratory where she'd worked before she left the Corporits.

Would the door open with Becky Quinn's card?

She slid it through the monitor—the door snapped open. She slipped inside and dropped to the floor so they couldn't see her through the glass panel.

It was like being in a cocoon. All sound was blocked from the corridor and the lab was silent as a tomb. She closed her eyes, waited for her breathing to slow down.

When she finally looked around, the first thing she saw was the disintegration chamber and the snake-like conveyor belt that wound its way through the room. The now motionless belt passed through each cubicle where other doctors like Zoe would dissect peoples' organs, ferret out usable tissue, and toss dead tissue away for destruction. After they finished carving up the different body parts, everything would be tossed onto the moving conveyor belt, carried to the large chamber for disintegration.

Tears flooded Zoe's face. She had never wanted to ever see this laboratory again. She and Laya had escaped from this very spot, and this was the place where Nathan Quinn and Seka Joraine had been vaporized.

Sobs tore at her chest. She cried and cried until there were no more tears.

Andrew! He would need her information—need the location and what she'd seen in the central control room. Zoe stood and peeked through the small window to see outside the lab.

No one there.

She stepped out into the corridor, listened for a few moments before heading for the exit door she'd used earlier. She slipped the card into the slot. The door opened slowly and then closed behind her. She stared down the stairwell—a search laser was starting its run up the exit staircase, looking for intruders.

She would have to work her way down, get out before the laser could trap her.

The light was inching up slowly, moving at a leisurely pace. At least they weren't looking for her yet. She hurried down as the light moved up.

It was getting closer and closer.

She wasn't going to make it.

Zoe fumbled slipping the card through a third-level door— it had no sooner snapped shut than she saw the search beam glow through the peephole. She turned around and walked into the main rotunda. It was very quiet.

Then she heard the *click-click-click-click* she'd heard earlier.

She peeked around a tank. Coming down the aisle was a stream of spider drones, heading right towards her.

Oh, my god!

She'd seen these small poisonous drones before, knew they injected paralyzing venom that killed within seconds.

She was mesmerized as she watched their shiny metal exoskeletons and their large ant-like eyes move towards her. They never slowed or sped up—they just formed uniform straight lines like a disciplined army with orders to march, capture, kill!

Click-click-click-click.

They would be on top of her in a moment.

172

She leaped up and dropped carefully into a tank filled with a floating child. She drew her legs up and squeezed inside, trying not to slosh. Right before she ducked under the fluid in the tank, she could hear the guards talking on the floor above.

"What's got the drones moving?"

"Hell, it could be a rat wandering around. We have them all over the place."

"Those spider drones are little killers, aren't they? Good thing we only use them on the third floor. I'm sure as hell not working around them."

"What are you afraid of?"

"I've seen those little fuckers get messed up. They destroy everything and anything in their path."

Click-click-click-click.

Zoe's heart echoed in the icy liquid solution—almost viscous, it smelled rank. The arms of the child kept clutching her into a deadly embrace, pulling her closer to it while its eyeless sockets stared at her.

Silent screams echoed in her brain.

Got to get out of here!

Got ... to ... get ... out.

She pulled away from the child and onto her knees. The skeletal arms tightened around her. She pulled her mouth out of the solution, heard the drones moving away.

She tore the child's arms off of her neck and climbed back out of the tank and onto the floor. Liquid dripped all around her while she limped to the exit door. She dropped her ident-card, and kept dropping it again and again.

Click-click-click-click.

They were coming back.

When she pushed the card through the slot, it refused entry. Too wet to register the signal.

She used her shaking fingers like a squeegee and put the ident-card through again.

"Open up. Open up. Please open up."

Click-click-click-click. Click-click-click-click.

The sound was almost deafening.

The door snapped open; Zoe rushed through and pushed it shut.

Click-click-click-click.

They were marching up and down the sealed door.

Chapter 35

Safe house

When Zoe started out for the Organ Harvesters complex, she hadn't dared hope for survival. Hope would only feed her fears and make her misstep.

And the reality?

She'd almost been done in by creepy spider drones in a venomous attack. The fact that she was still breathing seemed like a miracle to her.

In her soaking wet clothes and shoes, she sloshed towards the transpod. Even in the open air, she knew she smelled noxious and disgusting. But her luck held out—no one else was at the station at 3:00 AM.

Waiting for the pod to arrive, she tried to block out the vision of the doomed child that had been packed into a tank she'd been forced to share. The skin and muscles of its legs and arms had been stripped away. And yet, it felt alive to her—sentient enough to want Zoe to hold it.

Maybe that was her imagination. She tried to tell herself that, but no matter how hard she tried, she knew that child sensed Zoe's presence and it wanted to be loved.

It left her feeling empty.

Once in the transpod, riding back to the safe house, Zoe was shocked to see her skin was not only shriveled, it had an orange tint, probably from the preservative in the tank.

At her transpod stop, she saw no one until she left the station. From a distance she could see some people starting to take to the streets, leaving for early shifts.

She hurried back to the safe house, stripped off her clothes, and threw them away in a bin marked for disposables. With no shower in the unit, she had to wash herself from the small sink in the kitchen area. The orange tint lessened, but she still felt dirty even after she'd finished her attempts to clean up.

It was noon when Zoe opened her eyes, blinded by the harsh light. She'd only had four hours of sleep. After returning from the Organ Harvesters she'd remained in bed wide awake—too shaken to drift off.

Now she was exhausted, every part of her ached. She stretched to ease the pain, but was overcome by the realization that she was still alive.

It made her smile—she'd not only survived, she had the information that Andrew needed.

* * *

Andrew's Potter's Apartment

Andrew and Jin lay in each other's arms. She raised her head and looked at the face of her sleeping lover. She couldn't believe she'd finally found someone she could love forever.

Melik was out of town on business, at least that's what he'd said. Jin suspected he was probably with the red headed woman whose picture was in his locked desk drawer.

She quietly slid out of bed and went into the bathroom. She wanted to sing as she stepped into the shower and the warm water rushed over her hair, her body. She smiled when Andrew slipped in behind her. His warm hands slid across her thighs, ran across her belly, exploring. Whirling into his arms, she rubbed her breasts across his chest. He grabbed onto her and lifted her until she could wrap her legs around his waist. They kissed slowly, deeply, lips buried in each other.

* * *

When they were finished dressing, Andrew looked at this lovely woman, studied her long, dark hair, her eyes that looked at him with such radiance. If only he could forget about Defys, elections, CICs, planning, plotting. He only wanted to be with her.

He pulled her into his arms, then pulled her back into the bathroom. He ran the shower water, and said. "We have to talk."

"I hate talking. I'd rather make love to you ... that's what showers are for." She smiled up at him.

He pulled her closer. "Not today. Today, we hope the water will muffle our words so no one will hear what we say to each other. This is very important."

"I don't want to hear it, but I'm listening."

"Melik knows about us."

Jin's eyes widened. "Are you sure?"

"He kidnapped me, wrapped my head so I couldn't see him, and put me through the wringer."

"Are you sure it was him?" She held him at arm's length. "Did he hurt you?"

"Not really. I wasn't supposed to know who he was, but one of the goons who snatched me blurted out his name."

"Melik can be vicious." Jin's dark eyes were large with fear. "I know for a fact he's done some awful things to his enemies."

"I think it would best if we didn't see each other for a while."

"No, Andrew, don't say that." Tears ran down her cheeks. "I can't lose you."

He hugged her to him. "Listen, this is a critical time. All of us have a role to play. If any part of the election is screwed up, we're all finished."

"Not finished," she said. "Maybe delayed ... but not finished."

"It's taken years of planning and hard work to gather the Defys, to make people realize that if we don't take back our world, we're all going under." He took hold of her shoulders and looked deeply into her eyes. "It's now or never."

"I guess I just don't see it happening."

"Look, Jin. Our candidates have to win the election. But that's not all."

"What do you mean?" she looked puzzled.

"If we can bring down one of the most influential Corporits ... the one who seems to pull the strings not only here in Sanfrancorp, but worldwide ... don't you see, the whole Corporit structure would start to unravel."

"One person?" she said.

"Emory Dutton, CEO of the Medi-Progs, holds everything in his grip. It's all an integral part of the Organ Harvesters."

"Explain it to me. I don't see why organs for transplanting make the big difference."

Andrew went into his kitchen and filled two cups of corpcaf for them and brought them back to the bathroom.

"No one wants to die."

She smiled at him. "Well, that part I get." She reached for one of the cups, took a sip before holding it between her palms.

"Emory Dutton controls all the organs and their distribution," he said. "Not only that, he has organ depository satellites all over the globe. The complex in Sanfrancorp is the mother ship for all of them.

"How did he get to be so powerful?" she asked.

"By lying, cheating, blackmailing people in power who will do anything to stay alive," he said. "They either did what he wanted, whatever he asked, or they didn't get the body replacements they needed to survive."

Andrew could see from the look on her face that she was beginning to see the entire picture.

"It goes even deeper," he said. "What about the medicines you need to fight off a disease, or the vaccinations to keep you from becoming ill? Dutton could make sure you stayed ill because, I know for a fact, Pharmcorp's CEO is in Dutton's pocket. Most all of them are."

"It's hard to believe, Andrew. Can one man control so much of what happens on the planet?"

178

"Most people find it hard to believe, but he's pretty damn clever. Any opponents, or protestors find themselves donating their bodies and their organs whether they want to or not." Andrew took her hand. "And as long as he has the CAPOs there to carry out every single order he gives, the only way around it is to become a Noncorp."

"That's why Dutton hates the Quinns, hates my family," she said. "They've stood in his way for decades."

"And why he makes sure the populace is constantly terrified by nonexistent terrorists that are supposed to be taking over the Corporits' space. If the people find out the truth, the Corporits are going down."

"I guess we have to get the CIC's new candidates elected," Jin said with a sad smile.

"I can't do that and worry about you," Andrew said, taking her hand. "I have to know you're safe."

She set her cup on the sink and slid into his arms. "This is going to be the hardest thing I've ever done."

Chapter 36

CAPO Facility

George Potek sat at his desk sipping his corpcaf. He was doing his early morning scrolling through the reports of his investigative staff's review of Andrew Potter:

Request Order #1166 by Emory Dutton, CEO, Medi-Prog.

The reports and log-ins piqued Potek's interest.

It looked as though Emory Dutton was right. The robotics doctor *was* up to something. He'd definitely been eluding CAPO observation—and for a long time. It wasn't a question of why, but rather, who gave a damn anymore except Dutton?

Potek was agitated. He'd been having trouble sleeping and his unhappiness and sense of isolation were starting to affect his appetite—he'd begun to lose too much weight. He knew if he allowed himself to continue with this sense of alienation he would be in real trouble. He didn't have to look far to figure out why he had begun to decline.

Lately every single time Dutton called him into his office, he made sure Potek left feeling small, unimportant, useless, and a damn fool. And the last time when the CEO read the riot act to him—which he had begun to do on a daily basis—Potek hung back and said to himself, what his father used to say to him:

There will be consequences.

Potek thought, *CEO Emory Dutton. There will be consequences.*

What had been the final insult? When Dutton dinged him via the CAPO board, threatening Potek's job, threatening to turn him into a buck private marshal. That had pushed him over the edge: He wasn't about to forget that.

It was then the iciness of indifference he'd felt to both Dutton and his own situation rolled into something else.

Potek wanted revenge.

A buck private marshal, my ass. We'll see about that.

He would be damned if he was going to tell the big man anything more than he absolutely must.

It's time for Dutton to get a taste of what it's like to play in the dirt with the rest of us.

No more free passes.

When the alert came that Becky Quinn had signed into the Organ Harvesters complex at 1:00 AM, Potek knew he was onto something pretty damn important. And Dutton would have loved that piece of information. A good reason to bring in the Quinns for questioning.

Not on your life. Emory Dutton would never hear a word about it.

There will be consequences.

* * *

Argaret's Home

Hani Singer, Olga Yammo, and Podes Diaz were having a breakfast together. Not in a restaurant. It was in Argaret Charles' soundproof penthouse.

It had been difficult to get them together without attracting attention. Elections were about to occur and they all knew every step they took was being monitored by the CIC's internal police staff —which wasn't even supposed to exist—plus the CAPOs. But Argaret owned a huge building in Sanfrancorp. Because of her political influence, and her family wealth, she was on a very long leash and few of the policecorps ever caused her any problems.

"I see Mitchell Payette wasn't invited," Olga said to Argaret.

"It's my breakfast. I'll invite whom I want."

182

The Spaniard, Podes Diaz was looking as handsome as ever, Argaret thought. His dark wavy hair and flashing eyes always made her groin light up. She might be pushing fifty, but she wasn't dead yet. But that was secondary. He was one of the most creative thinkers she knew. She'd worked hard behind the scenes to make sure he came to the attention of nominating committee members—*supposedly* impartial groups chosen from Corporit communities at random.

But this time was different. Argaret and others had managed to infiltrate nominating committees with committed Defys. In the end, the three others at the table had been chosen to run for election along with incumbent members of the CIC, plus Mitchell Payette.

Argaret was also sure the three other people at the table were chosen to be on the slate of candidates because they were well-to-do Corporits. Payette and his backward way of thinking was a part of it only for show—a gift to Alan Fiss.

"Shall we eat and talk?" Argaret asked.

They all moved to the chafing stations in the large dining room. Dishes in hand, some opted for eggs, some for French toast. Everyone had a special cup of corpcaf, provided by Argaret's family corporation.

When they had almost finished eating, Argaret asked, "Are any of you satisfied with the existing CIC and its governing performance?"

Silence.

No one at the table responded.

"The members of this CIC have held their positions for many, many years," Argaret said. "And you can be sure not one of them is anxious to give up that realm of influence."

"Why should they want to? With all the perks it makes it easier to ignore the worsening of climate change conditions," Olga said.

"Or famine," Hani called out.

"And drought," Podes added.

"Yes." Argaret dabbed her lips with a napkin and set it on the table. "And if we don't get those idiots out of office ... things will only get worse."

"They have the upper hand," Hani said. "The populace believes that terrorists are responsible for everything that's wrong with the world."

Olga's face turned a fiery red. "I don't believe that. Not *everyone*. You must have heard of the Defys."

They all nodded.

"How many of you belong to that group?" Argaret asked, looking at each of them, then said, "Forget I asked that. However, let me just say, that group is a lot more powerful than any of you realize."

"What good are the Defys if they remain hidden?" Podes said. "People have to wake up and take control of their lives. Now!"

Olga stood. "Podes is right. I'm a Defy. If I die for letting you know that ... then that's the chance I'll take. It's time to speak up. Time to be heard." Then she plopped down with a what-have-I-done look on her face.

Hani stood. "It's way past time. I'm a Defy, too."

Both Podes and Argaret stood. "Yes," they both said, looking at each other.

"I take it then, Mitchell Payette isn't one of us?" Olga looked directly at Argaret and when she received a nod of agreement, stood up again, smiled widely, and reached out to the group.

They all grasped hands.

Chapter 37

THE DOMES

Asher Wind Storm stood between the rows of corn stalks filled with the ripening ears. He ran his fingers through the silken tassels and laughed. Nothing made him happier than walking through thriving plant life in the domes. It brought back treasured memories of his mother and father who had originally designed the huge vivariums to save all life on Earth.

He continued through many of the huge food domes that spread across what used to be wasteland. Wolf trotted close to him, searching for any signs of possible trouble.

Soon they were surrounded by groves of orange trees covered in clusters of perfumed flowers. Storm studied the beauty of these plants. It was inspiring to be able to grow flora at any time of the year within the domes. These vivariums not only fed people's stomachs, but allow them to inhale an aroma of something indefinable—something that fed their souls.

Being here in the domes always brought peace and joy to the Marcopian Indian mystic. He began to play his panpipes and the music lifted and floated around him. The sun felt warm on his back and he was happy as he walked into Tabo's encampment, his music announcing his arrival.

The food that had been provided for Tabo's people was beginning to strengthen them. The oozing sores that had covered their skin had almost healed and there was laughter echoing everywhere.

* * *

Tabo watched the tall Indian approach. The wolf had the same yellow eyes as the man and they shared a power Tabo could not grasp. The wolf was alert to every movement of not only the Indian but all of Tabo's people. It watched everything and everyone.

The Indian continued to make strange sounds with an instrument that Tabo had never seen before coming to the domes. The sounds made him feel safe and happy.

His tribe had migrated to the large bushes in the dome. He was told they held oranges, and those were bees flying in and out of the blossoms.

At first his tribe was worried when some of the insects became angry and some of the people were stung. But now the bees mostly seem to hang in the air or they flew in slow, lazy circles visiting the flowers. Seeing them fly also brought a strange sense of peace and quiet.

Storm said, "I see you like these plants."

Tabo smiled and looked into the eyes of the Indian. He sensed an ancient wisdom and strength emanating from deep within—it seemed to radiate from the man's bones.

The Indian knew many things. That too, made Tabo feel safe.

When he took hold of the hand offered by Storm, visions clouded Tabo's mind. He remembered his life from the time when he was very small. He even remembered the stories his father told him about living on land where there was snow on the ground every day. How his father and his followers left one day because of tales he'd heard about the warmth of a land near a large body of water.

When they arrived, even before Tabo was born, there was no snow, but his people were outcasts everywhere they went. Tabo remembered his father telling the stories of how no one wanted them.

The tribe wasn't allowed in the city and they had to move farther and farther away until all they had was the desolation and ugliness of the pits created by the dumped garbage from the big city.

Tabo was born into hopelessness. He always lived with anger and the need to raid anywhere he and his tribe could find food. His biggest rival was Godan. The man his father said was his brother.

Storm withdrew his hand and Tabo's visions melted away.

"We have never worked with the land," Tabo said.

The silence was heavy without the music. Storm said, "The world of the domes will shelter you, and when you start to dig and care for all the life around you, you will be filled with hope."

"How?"

"Others will teach you what is necessary, what you need to know. There are three other communities of Aughts in these domes. They work the corn fields and the wheat. You will tend the orange trees, or you can join them or live apart, as you choose.

Three of the children walked up to the wolf. They reached out their hands—the wolf sniffed each in turn and let them run their fingers through his fur.

"No one will turn you away from here, Tabo. You are welcome. We need you ... you need us. We will all come together and love the land."

Tabo knew this man who loved the land spoke only the truth.

For the first time in his life, he felt hope.

Chapter 38

SANFRANCORP

WE WILL NOT GIVE IN TO THE TERRORISTS
VOTE!
BRING BACK THE CIC TEAM THAT HAS KEPT YOU
SAFE!

The announcement came with a roar of static and a blast of sound that had been nonstop for most of every day for the past week.

Melik Bacha wanted to climb out of his skin. He couldn't even enjoy a peaceful luncheon with his sister, Marinda, in her luxurious apartment.

"I'm sick of hearing your name tossed out everywhere I go. All day long!" he said.

"But the big day is really soon. Can't take chances on losing." She patted his hand like he was a two-year-old.

"Cut it out, sis. We've been going through this bullshit ever since I can remember. I may be the youngest in the family, but I grew up on this political babble."

His sister looked worried. "There's talk we might be thrown out of office by a bunch of newcomers with radical ideas."

TERRORISTS ARE AMONG US ... THE CIC WILL
PROTECT YOU ... ADAM FISS, CEDRA CRESTING,
MARINDA BACHA ... YOU KNOW THESE PEOPLE ... GARY
BLICK, ARGARET CHARLES ... THEY HAVE BEEN YOUR
SHIELD AGAINST DISASTER

"What newcomers? Those losers running against you? What a pathetic bunch." He picked up his chicken salad sandwich and took a big bite out of it.

"Maybe so, but the Defys are probably behind the people who want to replace us and those candidates are growing strong. The people could vote us out of office."

"Our company employees will vote for who we tell them, to or they'll find themselves out of a job and tossed out of Sanfrancorp," Melik said. "You've got nothing to worry about."

"The one thing we haven't been able to change is the voting laws," she said. "Votes are still not our corporate property ... they say we have no influence with the outcome."

"Voting should be eliminated. Stupid idea giving people choices."

Marinda laughed. "We're working on it."

"What happened to your boy-toy?" Melik said. "He's usually here wandering around. I haven't heard a peep out of him."

"I got tired of him." Marinda's features hardened. "He thought he could say anything he wanted. He forgot who was in charge."

"Don't tell me you've had him tanked at the Organ Harvesters," he said, laughing. "He won't come back with a better attitude that way. In fact he won't come back at all."

"No! He'll just have to do real work from now on." She gave him an evil stare. "You're starting to sound more and more like Emory Dutton every day."

"Well, he knows how to run a corporation that has clout." Melik finished his sandwich and wiped his mouth. "Meeting with him once a week has taught me a lot."

"A lot of what? I'm not sure that's such a good thing. He's an obnoxious bastard." She took a sip of her tea and thought a moment. "How are you and Jin doing?"

"Not too well. I think she's having an affair with Andrew Potter."

"The Chief of Robotics?"

"That's the one." Melik didn't want to discuss his marriage with his sister, or anyone else, for that matter.

"Are you sure?" she pressed. "How serious is it?"

MEMBERS OF THE CIC ARE PROTECTING YOU FROM TERRORISTS ... DON'T CHANGE NOW ... THESE ARE YOUR PEOPLE ... THEY HAVE ALWAYS FOUGHT FOR YOU ... FISS, CRESTING, BACHA, BLICK, CHARLES ... A WINNING TEAM

"Can't they stop?" Melik stood and rushed to the window. Even though he knew the sound was coming from speakers on the top of buildings all over Sanfrancorp, he kept looking down at the streets.

"Sit down!" his sister ordered. "Still the bratty kid you've always been."

"Oh, shut up!"

Marinda's voice became soft and pleasing. "I've been wanting to ask you if you could perhaps get Jin to do a favor for me. After all, she is my sister-in-law."

"Why don't you ask her yourself?" He moved back to his chair and plopped down.

"I thought it would sit better coming from you."

He looked up at his sister. "Look, all she and I are doing is fighting. I don't think she'll do anything for me."

"Maybe if you'd stop sleeping with every woman who tosses her ass at you, the two of you would get along much better."

"So you're a marriage counselor now?"

"You listen to me, you little idiot. She's a Quinn. A Quinn! If you treat her badly, you could end up in real trouble. In fact, our whole family could end up with problems that I don't even want to think about—and all because you couldn't keep your pecker in your pants or speak with a civil tongue."

"What are you talking about?"

"Think!" she said. "What if Quinn and his wife—that whole Quinn contingency—start complaining about our hospital instruments and pushes for one of the startups? They could put us out of business. Are you getting the picture?"

"I hadn't thought about that," he said.

"Well, think." She put a hand on his. "And while you're thinking about that, maybe you might ask Jin if she could plug my name for reelection? I mean, just *my* name. There's no reason I should have to go down with a sinking ship."

"By sinking ship, you mean the other present members on the CIC board?"

"Now you're beginning to get the picture ..."

Her last words were drowned out.

TERRORISTS WILL WIN ... THEY WILL INVADE YOUR HOME ... KILL YOU

Chapter 39

HOSPITAL-CORP
Storage Area M

Becky and Tris Quinn looked at the large crowd of people that had squeezed into the abandoned basement morgue in the bowels of the hospital. They'd all come during the lunch hour when there was massive movement in the hospital and people generally were out of their departments.

The Quinns had used this room many times in the past for holding secret meetings. Everyone present knew this section of the hospital had been a part of the Pathology Department—that service had been moved to an upper floor, along with the coroner's labs. The area was now a designated storage space.

Tris Quinn stood and picked up a microphone:

"Thank you for coming today. I'll cut right to it since everyone knows why we're here: Blatant medical malpractice. People have died because of one man's decadent leadership and our compliance, which allows it to continue."

There was a grumble of dissatisfaction.

"The VMAS patch, which was suppose to stabilize the horrific disease that has plagued our populations for the last twenty years, was actually an accelerator, causing people to die in terrible pain. Thousands are dead because of the irresponsible action on the part of CEO Emory Dutton."

Someone raised his hand. Tris pointed to him.

"Are you sure this rests at his doorstep?"

"I'm sure all of you will remember the day when everyone in medicine was called to a special meeting for the announcement of a vaccine to prevent VMAS."

Most everyone nodded.

"If you'll recall, at that time Emory Dutton announced that the Medi-Progs would also provide the stabilizing patch for those who were already infected."

There was a low assenting murmur all around the room.

"This solution was hailed around the globe as a cost-effective means of containing this disease for those who were already infected and unable to have the vaccine. As we all know, the existing stabilizer had been called unacceptable for the population at large because of its prohibitive cost."

Tris banged his fist on the table.

"Three days after the start of the preventive program, dead bodies were piling up in the streets across the globe."

"He's been lying to us all along," the Chief of Medicine said, jumping to her feet. "It's despicable!"

Tris looked at his watch. "We have to end this very quickly so we can blend in with the lunch crowd returning to work."

There was a murmur of agreement.

Becky stood, looked at each and every doctor.

"I propose that Quinn Foundation present a motion to the CIC on behalf of the Medi-Prog physicians in Sanfrancorp. Emory Dutton needs to be held accountable for his crimes against humanity. It's time we stopped this madness."

* * *

Adam Fiss's Home

The Supreme Interrogator hadn't slept for two nights. Each night he'd had to move into the spare room to get away from his wife's complaints. And she was right. All he did was toss and turn or wake up in a cold sweat from horrible nightmares where he was forced to walk through landscapes filled with bloody and mutilated bodies. When he jolted awake, he was shaking.

Tonight he ambled into his study, circled the desk, and pulled out his chair. He stared at the paper folders stacked in front of him, something he rarely saw anymore. All the paperwork covered background checks of three of the candidates, information he'd had his assistant dig out. These were the people who were threatening to unseat him or others on the CIC. He could have the reports on the telelink but he didn't want anything traced back to him.

Olga Yammo was the candidate who worried him the most. Rumor was that she was hoping to unseat him as the Chief Interrogator.

Such an ordinary-looking woman, but she was a much respected doctor and one with a big mouth, very critical of the way he ran the CIC. She'd accused him of taking money for favorable decisions and special treatment to certain Corporits and their families.

Of course what she said was true, but Adam couldn't afford to have the populace aware of it. Recently, she published a news bulletin and volunteers handed out copies of it in the malls and at transpod stations. He'd seen one of those flyers and there was nothing in it that was ever going to make him shine. It must have cost her a fortune.

No one knew the real effect it was having, but News-div publicity assured him it was just hot air. Adam wasn't that sure.

He liked his life and all the privileges he had. He would *have* to do something to show his dedication to justice and leadership. Something he'd never been asked to do before. He needed to create a platform that would demonstrate his interest in the populace and their well-being.

He pulled out a pen from the bottom drawer of his desk, scribbled lines on a piece of paper.

Most of the complaints that the CIC was asked to act on were in some way a result of the Medi-Progs. Emory Dutton's medical programmer's corporation was constantly being accused of unethical treatment and favoritism.

More and more facts were coming to light about Organ Harvesters and its hold on the CEOs who used its services. It was like the rings in the pond after a pebble hit the surface. Dutton controlled it all and everything Dutton did impacted someone else, and on and on.

Maybe it was time to rethink his relationship with Emory Dutton.

* * *

MEDI-PROG FACILITY
CEO's Office

Emory Dutton didn't like the look on his assistant's face as he ambled into his office. Usually the young woman had a big, stupid grin on her face as though each morning was a special gift. No syrupy "good morning" today as Dutton came through the door.

The first thing he saw—in the middle of his desk—was a subpoena issued by the CIC. Dutton was to appear before the committee first thing tomorrow morning.

Tomorrow!

"What?" he said out loud to his empty office.

He immediately picked up a telelink and impatiently dialed the CIC offices.

An office assistant picked up the call. "Good morning. May I help you?"

"Damn right. I need to speak to Adam Fiss ... right now!"

"May I ask who is calling?"

"Don't mess around with me, little girl. Put Adam Fiss on ... now!"

"I'm sorry. But I will need your name, sir."

"Tell him Emory Dutton is calling."

"One moment, please."

Dutton felt like he was jumping out of his skin—his heart was pumping furiously and he was panting for air.

After a few minutes, the assistant was back on the line. "I'm afraid Mr. Fiss is not available at the moment. Is there a message I can take to him?"

"You bet your ass there is. Tell him I'm on my way to his office. And he'd better be there when I arrive."

"Sir—"

Dutton hung up.

Bette Golden Lamb

Chapter 40

Emory Dutton's face was hot—red spots flashed before his eyes as he picked up the subpoena and started to tear it up. But he didn't dare.

His first thought was to call for his limo—drive to the CIC offices. He needed to move, needed action to stop his restless fury from pushing him into doing something stupid. He couldn't just sit around here like some passive fool and wait for his driver to get his ass in gear.

He needed to get going now.

He stomped out of his offices, took the elevator down, and walked out the front door. For a moment he was confused. He'd never traveled by the transpod system. It would have been the quickest route to the CIC offices, but he wasn't even sure how to get to the station. Instead, he moved in the direction of the ambulated walkway. He knew where that was.

At the entrance, he followed the crowd jockeying for positions on the automated belt that circled and transected the city. People were pushing, elbowing, and shoving him around.

"Hey, cut it out," he said to one woman who pushed him out of the way.

"Learn to move a little faster, old man."

He was stunned. "You better watch who you're talking to."

She turned to stare at him. "Yeeeeeah, and what are you gonna do about it?"

He wanted to slap that sarcastic smile off her face, but he stopped himself and turned away from her.

"I thought so." Soon she moved to an exit off the belt and was out of sight.

He squeezed his hand into a fist. His nails dug deep into his palm.

* * *

Forty minutes later he pushed through the doors of the CIC building.

A young, attractive female receptionist walked up to Dutton. Women like her were hired by the largest corporations. They were usually dressed in suggestive tight dresses, just the way this one was.

"Can I help direct you, sir?"

She didn't know who he was. Dutton wasn't used to being treated in an off-handed manner. The experience on the ambulated walkway had been enough of that for one day. He wasn't just anyone and people usually knew that, knew who he was anywhere, anyplace, anytime. And they took care of him.

"I'm here to see Chief Interrogator Fiss."

The woman's eyes narrowed. "Is he expecting you, sir?"

"He damn well better be," Dutton blurted.

"Sir, Chief Fiss only sees people by appointment. If you don't have one, we'll be happy to accommodate you, help you to make one ... but otherwise you'll have to leave."

Dutton slapped her face. The red imprint of his hand remained smeared across her cheek.

She hardly reacted except to call out, "Security!"

Dutton knew his mouth was hanging open as two private policemen hurried up to him. Each one grabbed an arm. "You'll have to leave, sir."

He spat the words out to the woman. "You tell Chief Fiss I'm here! Now!"

A crowd had gathered around the scuffle. He could hear their excited mumbling. The police dragged him down a long corridor where they opened the door and threw him inside.

"You'll pay for this!" he shouted at the closing door.

Dutton yanked out his telelink and punched in Potek's number.

* * *

The two policemen opened the door and George Potek stepped up to Dutton—he was sitting in a chair looking exhausted. His tie was loose, hanging at the neck, and sweat mapped the armpits of his suit jacket.

Dutton looked at him with eyes that flashed like bolts of lightning. "So you finally decided to show up, Potek?"

"I came as quickly as I could, sir."

Don't like seeing the other side of things, do you?

"Well, it wasn't quick enough."

"I'm doing the best I can," Potek said.

"Get me up to Chief Fiss's office right now. Do you hear me, you little slug?"

"He won't see you without an appointment." Potek moved in closer. "There's nothing I can do about it, sir."

"The CAPOs have no control here?"

"No, sir. The CIC has its own private security and they don't recognize any other law enforcement agency since an assassination attempt five years ago."

Potek offered an arm to help Dutton up. He pushed it away.

"Are you saying I can't see Adam Fiss unless he grants me an appointment?" Dutton struggled to his feet.

"That's true, sir," Potek said.

"Listen to me, you stupid fuck. You get me in to see the Chief Interrogator or you're out on your ass." Dutton started for the door. "He can't treat me like this. That son-of-a-bitch is not getting away with this."

"Yes, sir." But the CAPO Commander had to work very hard not to smile.

Chapter 41

Safe House

Someone was pounding on the door.

Zoe put down her cup of tea and tiptoed to see who it was.

Dammit! Who can that be?

If it was the CAPOs they would have broken it down by now. The pounding was letting up, but it still continued.

This will attract attention. I have to open it.

Holding her breath she unlatched the door. Jin Bacha flung it open, almost knocking Zoe down. She ran into the room and Zoe quickly closed the door and locked it.

"Jin. What's the matter?"

"Melik is going to kill me."

Zoe was stunned. "Are you sure?"

Jin collapsed in the only chair in the small unit. "He sent his sister Marinda to talk to me."

"What happened?" Zoe sat on the end of the unmade bed and reached for Jin's hand.

"She said Melik knew I was having an affair with Andrew Potter and her brother was coming for me."

"Do you really think he would do that? Kill you, when a divorce would be so easy and the civilized thing to do?" Zoe poured a cup of tea for Jin. When she reached for it, her hands were shaking.

"You don't know Melik ... he isn't civilized. He wants what he wants when he wants it, and he has a violent temper. He's vicious if he thinks anyone has crossed him." Tears filled her eyes. "I'm his property. He once told me he would never let me go ... I would still be his, even if he only used me as a punching bag."

"Andrew might be able to stop him."

Jin shook her head. "Don't you understand? No one can stop him. Andrew and I can't even see each other until after the election ... can't take the chance. Melik's sister said—"

"Why did she even bother to warn you?"

"She's only thinking of her own campaign." Jin said. "I don't think headlines that scream across the buildings—**Marinda Bacha's Brother Murders Wife**—would do much for getting her elected."

At that moment more name-blasting static boomed out across the city.

WE WILL NOT GIVE IN TO THE TERRORISTS
VOTE!
BRING BACK THE CIC TEAM THAT HAS KEPT YOU
SAFE

"That noise is everywhere," Zoe said. "It's like the streets are screaming at us with their political blasts. And now it's day *and* night. I can't sleep."

Zoe watched Jin set her tea cup down. Lost in her own thoughts, Jin looked off to an unknown distance—"Hmmmmm."

"What?" Zoe asked, her voice edgy.

For a moment Jin didn't respond. Then she suddenly broke out laughing. She kept doing it until Zoe thought she would never stop.

"Would you mind letting me in on the joke?" Zoe said. "One minute you're terrified, and the next you're laughing your head off."

"Well, if I wasn't so shook up ... so panicked, I would have thought it was strange that Marinda would bother to interfere in our marriage in any way ... good or bad." Jin couldn't stop smiling. "She never even cared enough to show up at our wedding."

"Still, Melik is her brother."

"I can tell you ... no love lost there." Jin stood and moved to the small window. "If anything, they barely tolerate each other."

"I'm still not getting it," Zoe said.

Jin turned back to her. "It's a scam." Jin must have seen the confusion on Zoe's face. "In essence, she said she'd rein in Melik if I pushed her name on strip news as a first-rate candidate."

"Can you do that?" Zoe asked, smiling.

"Of course I can."

Jin walked back to her seat.

"That's not the question, Zoe."

"What is, then?"

"The big question," Jin said with a wide smile, "is will I do it?"

Bette Golden Lamb

Chapter 42

Robotics—Surgical Suite

Andrew couldn't stop smiling, thinking about Jin as he walked out of his office and headed for the Surgical suites.

"Goodnight," he said to Dutton's undercover spy. He could almost see the pheromones cued to match his personal tastes riding up and down her skin.

She had a perplexed look on her face every time he left. Andrew guessed this special Dutton treat expected him to lick her from head to toe.

No thanks. The day I can't out smart Emory Dutton is the day I'll pack it in.

He knew how to play a game of compliance. His ex-wife had made him an expert at that.

He was feeling pretty strong again and wanted to flex his regained muscle strength. His thigh wound was almost back to normal and his shoulder only jabbed at him every now and then. The special ointment Storm sent had accelerated healing, had done a great job of pushing his progress way beyond his expectations.

And there she was again ... Jin popping into his head.

In love, like he'd never been before.

He couldn't help thinking of how they were together. She was like a beautiful fresh flower covered in morning dew. The kind he saw when he visited Storm's Caplac Domes, where huge spreads of acres were filled with flowers.

He once asked Storm why he bothered growing flowers when food and so many other essentials were far more important.

Storm had laughed at him. Yes, laughed as though Andrew were a little boy with no common sense. "What would our planet be like without flowers and the bees that are drawn to them? Think of life without their beauty, their wild sensuality that stirs our imagination."

Right now Andrew could imagine a whole dome filled with Jins—lovely, beautiful, moist, inviting, and waiting for him.

Cut it out, man. You won't be good for anything if you keep this up.

Thinking of Storm's domes made Andrew think of Zoe again.

It had seemed as though she was a woman destined to die young. In fact, she had been about as close to death as anyone could possibly get and still be alive. Now, she too was healing, but with a new sense of reality. She'd been transformed from a consumer into a defender of the planet. He was proud of the new Zoe. Her dead husband, Elliott, would have been proud, too.

The information she'd brought to him after her visit to the Organ Harvesters was crucial. Now he understood the kinds of neural sequencing he would have to use to try to save anyone floating in one of those tanks. It was a definite gray area. He'd never seen or heard of any of the people in the tanks returning to normalcy again. A trip to the tanks was always a one-way trip.

* * *

Andrew undressed quickly and stashed his clothes in one of the drawers in the pre-decontamination chamber. He was getting tired of always being the late one to these Defy meetings, but there was no way he could have left his office earlier without arousing suspicion.

Naked, he moved into the decontamination room. He tried without success to block out the horrible music the department provided. It was what they used to call Muzak in the elevators— boring, uninspiring, and dull—like so much of Corporit culture.

He was so deep in thought that the bacto-viral solution caught him off guard and some of it ended up in his mouth. He tried to spit it out, but the sensors didn't accept that kind of betrayal. The brushes came back and scrubbed his lips until he thought his mouth and gums would end up raw and bleeding.

"Son-of-a-bitch," he said out loud between swipes.

That's it. If I can't put this brain of mine to work and create a more humane body decontamination process, then my name isn't Andrew Potter.

At last, he was freed after the sensors evaluated not only every inch of his body, but every crevice. The light flashed green and a cybernetic voice said: "You may now enter the surgical suite, Dr. Potter."

Fuck you very much.

* * *

C called out to Andrew as he stepped stark naked into Robotics Theater one. "Ah-huh, you finally made it."

Andrew raised an eyebrow. "I know we don't use our real names, but I can think of one I'd like to call you. But everyone would then know who you are."

"Go ahead," C said.

D chimed in, "That's enough foreplay. This is probably our last get-together before the election."

B had a deadly stare. "We may all be naked, but I want to check everyone's ears to make sure there are no tiny hidden recorders. That sudden visit by the CAPOs last time shook me up."

They all checked each other.

"Satisfied," A said.

"Good enough."

They began opening the surgical trays and setting up the surgiclones for studying in case they had another CAPO visit.

B said to A, "Do we have anyone in News-Div to hit the building strips with info nailing Dutton for crimes against humanity? We need a person that people can focus on—that prick has more than earned it."

A said, "I think so."

Andrew hated to tell them about Ethan. "The one who would have been more than glad to step up is now residing in one of the harvesting tanks."

"Jeez," B said, "There but for the grace ..." He paused. "That could have been anyone of us."

"I know," C said. "We didn't sign up for this because it was the safe thing to do." He looked at Andrew. "The tanked one. Was that the man I suggested we approach?"

Andrew nodded.

"Damn," C said. "That's going to give me nightmares."

"Who's going to replace him?" B asked. "We need someone from News-div to get the word out to the whole city ... and it has to be on the voting day so it can't be shut down. It's an essential part of the plan."

"I'm hoping that it'll be done," Andrew said.

"That's not good enough," B said. "Dutton has to go down with crimes against humanity for that bogus stabilizer against VMAS."

"And Olga Yammo, Hani Singer, and Podes Diaz have to be elected," C said. "Or it's right back to the same old game of Corporit business as usual."

"All of this has been a leap of faith," Andrew said. "Our underground newspaper has been inundating the populace for two weeks solid."

"And so has the Corporit propaganda, blasting everyone in the city," D said

"We've grabbed onto everyone we can," Andrew said. "And we'll keep up the heat. It's three days from the vote. Two more days to inundate the populace."

"I don't think I can take another six years of those CIC bastards," D said.

They all nodded.

Chapter 43

AUGHT TERRITORIES

Godan and ten of his trusted warriors roamed through the deserted lands of Tabo's tribe. He remembered the night Tabo came to him and threw down his knife as a sign of peace. When Godan had awakened the next day, he thought it was a dream. But the man who was supposed to be his brother and his worst enemy was really gone. This land was deserted.

Godan squatted and touched the dry, gravelly soil. He dug his nails in, let his fingers ride through its emptiness. Nothing was living in the ground, nothing above.

Yes, Tabo was gone.

Something hot coiled inside. Not the anger he usually felt. It was painful, like a knife being twisted inside. It not only made him feel strange, it made him sad and lonely. Tears ran down his cheeks.

He did not want to come here. He wanted to forget about his brother, but Tabo was haunting him.

He came to Godan each and every night when he closed his eyes and returned to the unknowable sleeping world. Godan hated that shadowy place filled with not only his enemies and fears, but with the strange beings that lived only there. In that darkness he was a coward, running from his attackers—he always woke up shaking and afraid.

When Tabo appeared in his dreams, he held out a hand in peace. "Do not be afraid."

"What do you want?"

Tabo's face was covered in scars from his battles as an Aught, but his eyes were ... calm. "Come with me, brother. It's time to leave."

Godan stood next to him and looked up at his face. "This is my home. I belong here."

"You will die here. Leave the emptiness of the garbage pits and find your way to the domes. Come! They will save you and your people."

Tabo had something around his neck. When Godan stepped closer, it was like the medallions he'd seen around the necks of many people when he raided the domes. An eye that looked like the powerful angry eye Godan had seen in the sky.

The sleeping world only confused him.

"Go away," Godan told his brother.

But Tabo would not leave the darkness. He returned to Godan every night.

He went to Tabo's country to stop the visions; he searched through the garbage tunnels, stood and listened for any sign of life. But the land was empty. All that remained were the bodies of the sick who had died.

* * *

NONCORP DOME TERRITORY

Asher Wind Storm had made a sacred promise to Zoe before she left for Sanfrancorp. He would help the Aughts. Give them a choice of survival or death. It had been hard to bring in Tabo and his followers. All of the Aughts killed much too easily and his anger towards Godan for the death of his dear friend Arina Marek burned deep within. They had murdered her. His heart could not find peace when he thought of the Aughts, especially Godan.

Storm sat in the center of his medicine wheel, his closest disciples surrounding him. They chanted together. Storm knew he had to purge himself of his hatred, his longing for revenge.

Today he had brought the stones that held the spirits of his mother and father, placed them in the center of the wheel. They made him feel connected. Safe. He looked to the sky.

We are all brothers and sisters.

Visions of Arina and her mutilated body centered around him—would not leave. He chanted and chanted. The visions did not change. Arina remained. Naked. Mutilated. Penetrated. Murdered.

We are all brothers and sisters.

Wolf stepped into the circle, lay down next to Storm. And as amber eyes met, a sense of peace returned and washed over the warrior. His boiling blood began to cool and he bowed to the wisdom of the Great Spirit in the universe.

"My brothers and sisters, it is a time of renewal. The Earth and the peoples of the world have suffered at the hands of the few. As the domes continue to spread across the land we must be ready to take back our land. We must be ready for deliverance."

Storm touched the stones that represented his mother and father. One on each side of him. He knew their spirits hovered near.

"For those who can accept the evolution of change, who can find their way back to an Earth healed and whole again, to a life that can be lived in dignity for all, they will be the survivors of a new world."

Storm opened his arms to the all. "Those who cannot, will perish."

The winds began to circle around the Earth. A whirl of dust spun around Storm and Wolf.

The eternal eye rose, blinked at the Earth.

* * *

Godan sat at the top of a mound. He looked across the landscape and watched a whirl of dust blow closer and closer until it spun above him.

The air turned cold and an eye hovered above Godan.

His men ran for the garbage pits and crawled inside.

Godan was empty. He had never felt this alone. He looked up at the eye. "If you want to kill me, kill me. I don't want to live anymore."

For an instant the cold air turned to frost, but then it warmed.

His mind spoke to him:

Come away from here, Godan. Leave this emptiness and join Tabo in the domes. Let your enemy become your soul mate.

Tabo will kill me.

He has asked you to come.

So he can kill me.

The dust whirled even faster. A tear fell from the sky.

You can be with your people forever in the domes. Together you can feel life grow under your fingers. You can know joy.

Joy? I don't know what that is.

You will learn.

The wolf that traveled with the Indian appeared out of nowhere. It slowly moved to Godan until it was at his side.

Godan touched its head, then ran his fingers through its fur. The wolf lay down next to him.

Chapter 44

Emory Dutton's Office

When Potek arrived at Dutton's office suite, the CEO was standing next to Astrid's desk in the reception area, waiting for him. It was obvious that the assistant was not only nervous, but very upset with Dutton standing over her. He'd probably been badgering her the whole time he was waiting.

"Get your ass in my office, Potek."

Potek followed Dutton inside and stood at attention. Dutton's eyes were bloodshot; he looked like he hadn't slept in days.

"Do you have any notion in that thick skull of yours how humiliating that was?" Dutton circled Potek. He looked like he was spilling viscous bile everywhere. "I have never been refused admittance to the Chief Interrogator. Adam Fiss will pay for this." Dutton looked at Potek. "Do you hear me?"

"Yes, sir, I hear you."

"I want to see him. Do you understand?"

"What would you like me to do, sir?"

"Well, I'd like you to strip the skin off his body and send him to hell."

"Sir, I don't think I can do that. The man is in charge of the CIC."

"I must see him, Potek. I must talk to him."

"Have you tried making an appointment, sir?"

"You sound like those idiots at his office. Am I some cretin off the streets? Am I some low-level nothing, like you?"

Potek felt his stomach clench. All he wanted to do was slap the CEO, kick him to the ground and beat the shit out of him.

215

"Sir, I respectfully submit, I couldn't even get an appointment to see the Chief Interrogator no matter what I did."

"Of course not. You're just a thug. But I'm not. *I* want to see him."

"I'll talk to his office."

Dutton's voice softened. "This is a critical time, Potek. If any of the people challenging the seated members win the election ... well, I'm in for a rough ride."

"I'll see what I can do, sir."

* * *

George Potek went back to his van and burst out laughing. He laughed so hard he could hardly grab a breath—tears ran down his cheek.

At that moment he was a teenager again, remembering his father being dragged away because he wouldn't give in to Emory Dutton. Potek never found out the particulars of the problem, no matter how hard he tried.

What had his father refused to do?

Potek had buried that last vision of his father for many years. What he never stopped forgetting was his mother and her sadness. She died not long after they took his father away. She just stopped eating and Potek knew she died from a broken heart.

He swore he would never depend on someone else. People brought you down. Potek would only do something where he could control his fate.

He became a CAPO and he never regretted it until recently when he began to think of his father again. Think of the last day he saw him. That, and the way Dutton had treated him.

It had taken years, but Potek finally realized he didn't like being treated as though he didn't exist.

There are consequences, Emory Dutton.

* * *

CIC Offices

Adam Fiss was steaming. That Emory Dutton would come to his offices and behave the way he did was totally unacceptable.

He picked up his telelink and set up a conference call with C.C., Marinda, Gary, and Argaret Charles. All of them were jumpy about the election. Even with all the constant publicity in their favor booming across Sanfrancorp, they were all running scared.

"Hi, all," the chief said.

Each responded.

"I have before me, initiated by Advocatecorp, a writ accusing CEO Emory Dutton of crimes against humanity."

Marinda Bacha responded without hesitation. "Are you kidding me?"

C.C.: "Which crime? The man's a walking horror story."

The Chief said dryly, "It states Dutton deliberately expedited VMAS by giving patients with the disease an accelerator patch that would medically kill them."

Gary Blick: "Who hired the Advocatecorps?"

Argaret Charles answered: "Undoubtedly it was the Quinn bloc. They're the only group of people with the courage to stand up to Dutton. What do you think, Adam?"

Adam Fiss let the question hang there for a moment. He finally said, "I have subpoenaed Dutton to appear tomorrow."

Marinda: "Why don't you bury it until after the election? Once things are back to normal, you know after all the opposition's hype is over and done with."

"Marinda," the chief said, "you know we can't do that. We can't ignore Advocatecorp. Also, every Defy—and I have to reiterate, we don't have an exact number of these Corporit rebels—would nail us. We'd go down with Dutton."

Argaret said: "Yes, that's true, Chief. We have to be what we're supposed to be."

Gary said with a chuckle, "And what is that?"

217

C.C. jumped in. "We are supposed to be the final arbiter of the Corporits. There is no other global law greater than ours. We have the ultimate power and we have to use it wisely. If this accusation is true, Dutton has solely, without sanction, committed a deliberate, heinous crime. He is responsible for the murder of huge numbers of people and must be held responsible."

* * *

Adam Fiss was being pushed into a corner. There was no doubt that he was complicit in setting up the tainted VMAS patch. Protecting Dutton was the only way he could save himself. His doctor had recently told him he would need an organ transplant in the near future. There was no kidding himself, Dutton was his best, maybe only chance for survival.

He remembered the conversation before Dutton created the VMAS accelerator.

The two of them were having dinner together. Dutton had initiated the get-together and they were dining at one of the few remaining twentieth-century plush establishments in Sanfrancorp.

Both were having strawberry tarts for dessert when Dutton said, "I think I have a way to drastically cut the population."

"As you've said *ad nauseam,* there's no doubt we have to shrink the growing number of people. The human habitat is being totally destroyed." Fiss loved these theoretical conversations. "We know that, but still, there are no real solutions to this dilemma."

"That's where you're wrong, Adam. I have one that's very doable."

"I can't imagine what you have in mind." Adam laughed so hard he almost choked on a glazed strawberry. This obviously wasn't going to be theoretical.

"We have a great medical breakthrough." Dutton said. "And you can't reveal this to anyone. Do you understand?"

"Dammit, do I look like some idiot. I know what a secret is."

Dutton took the last bite of his tart and leaned back in his chair, chewing slowly. "Of course you know VMAS has been a scourge all across the planet."

"Obviously, Emory. Stop treating me like an idiot. You might have noticed I never shake hands with anyone. Last thing I need is VMAS ... I don't take chances, no matter how they say you become infected."

Dutton smiled. "We have a vaccine for VMAS."

"What! Damn, that's fantastic!" Adam felt a great sense of happiness and well-being. He could cross that disease off the list of things he was afraid of. "That's great news. Why not blast it everywhere?"

Dutton had a strange look in his eyes. "It doesn't work on anyone who already has the disease. The people who are infected will continue to linger for six months or more, as they do now, using up our medical supplies and medical personnel's time and energy ... and cost us large sums of capital."

"Well, there's nothing to be done about that."

Dutton said, "Well, actually there is."

Fiss leaned halfway across the table. "What?"

"We'll make the vaccine announcement, advise that we have a cost-effective stabilizer for those already infected, and they are to be given simultaneously to the public within a three-day inoculation period."

"What happens to the infected people who get the stabilizer?" Adam finally sat back in his chair.

"Why, they receive a VMAS accelerator and they die within three days," Dutton said, waited a moment, then smiled.

* * *

"Chief?" Argaret said. "Do you hear me?"

"I'm sorry," Adam said, hating that memory. "Could you repeat your last question?" He could hear the grumble of the committee members. They'd all had enough of this conference call.

"Do you think the charge of crimes against humanity are true?" Argaret said.

"I've issued a subpoena. Dutton will appear here tomorrow for questioning," Adam said "We will find out then."

"Again, the day before the election?" Marinda asked.

"Yes."

Chapter 45

George Potek was following two of the candidates in the upcoming CIC election. No one had asked him to personally take charge of that detail, but his intuition was working overtime. He usually sent someone from his staff to do the tailing, but he needed to stay busy.

His hatred towards Dutton was eating into him. Like a poison, it was invading his thoughts every day until it was all he could think of. He hadn't had a decent night's sleep in weeks.

This morning, one of his staff had alerted him to a meeting between Marinda Bacha and Mitchell Payette. The information piqued his curiosity.

He didn't like the Bacha woman, or her family. They were always on his back, demanding special protection privileges and there was never a really good reason, or was there? Actually, being afraid that someone in the general populace would kill them, was a reasonable fear. And they wanted to enjoy an illusion of a safe, plush environment with some kind of bodyguard guaranteeing their continued life.

Potek eyed Bacha and Payette sitting in an upscale cafe. They were sipping coffee, but there was no sign of any food being brought to them.

Potek had already electronically bonded both of their telelinks. He sat in a CAPO hovervan and punched in the listening device on in his unit and eavesdropped:

"She'll do what I tell her," Marinda said.

"Why do you even care?" Mitchell said. "If you ask me, being on the CIC board is just a lot of work and no play."

She laughed. "And you're running because?"

"Why, for women, of course," he said. "Have you looked at my face, Marinda ... and I'm not young and engaging anymore. Who would want to go to bed with someone like me if I didn't have the juice to make it worthwhile?"

"But, Mitch, you could sit on one of the most powerful seats on the globe. I've been there for years and I love it. Believe me, power never grows old."

"Marinda, Marinda, Marinda. Who cares? Remember when it used to be great to be rich? You could go anywhere in the world, anytime. Lie on a beach, swim in the ocean."

"You can still do that."

"Sure. You can go to an oil-soaked stretch of sand they stopped cleaning up twenty years ago ... then drop into the garbage-filled ocean for a quick swim. Do you really think that's fun? Don't you get it? Nothing is beautiful anymore. The only thing good about politics is it makes it all a little less boring."

"Poor Mitchell, all that money and nowhere to spend it."

Potek watched them through the restaurant window. A server brought a platter full of what looked like pastries. Potek was too far away to be sure. The waiter also kept coming back to refill their coffee cups.

"Rumor has it that Emory Dutton has been subpoenaed. That's a delicious piece of gossip," Mitchell said.

Potek sat up in his seat and began to listen more closely.

"Yes. He's accused of committing crimes against humanity," Marinda said. "Who would think they'd ever dream of trying to nail *his* ass?"

"I didn't hear about that. That really is delicious. Crimes against humanity, huh?" he said. "What did he do?"

"He messed with the VMAS stabilizer," she said. "Made it a killer patch. You know ... he's a population control freak. Why bother to fix the planet when you can just cut down on the population?"

"It always made sense to me," he said, laughing. "I just don't want to be the one to go."

"Funny, how it always matters whose ox is being gored," Marinda said.

"He'll get away with it. No one gets to shit on Dutton's parade," Mitchell sounded sarcastic. "Who's the accuser?"

"Advocatecorp," her voice was almost in a whisper.

"Yeah, but who's the client?"

"The Quinn Foundation," she said.

"I should have known. They're the only ones who have ever had the balls to go to battle with Dutton ... and survive." There was a long pause. "Aw, he'll get off."

"You're probably right," Marinda said. "That's because no one really wants to mess with that man ... not with all those body parts stacked and waiting to be used to keep us alive."

"Brrr, let's not talk about it ... it gives me the shivers."

* * *

Potek sat tapping his finger on the dashboard in a strange rhythm.

So that's what the subpoena is about. Crimes against humanity.

No wonder Dutton was acting even crazier than usual, especially when Potek finally told him there was nothing he could do to get him in to see the Chief Interrogator.

Dutton actually picked up a chair and threw it at him.

Potek left his listening post—he'd heard enough from these two.

He decided to drop into a spa. A hot tub soak would make him feel even better.

But he couldn't stop grinning.

Oh, yes. There are consequences, Emory Dutton.

Bette Golden Lamb

Chapter 46

SAFE HOUSE

Zoe was tossing and turning. She couldn't seem to get comfortable. She hadn't shut down or drifted off to sleep all night. Thinking about the coming elections, had her excited and fearful.

She flung the covers aside and jumped up, walked to the window, looked out toward the east and the rising sun.

The streetlights were flicking out one by one. The city was waking, not yet fully stirring. She tried to see the sky beyond the city dome, but the glare from the news strips on the tops of all the buildings was a glittering distraction. The early morning quiet was disrupted by the renewed cacophony of propaganda:

**VOTE FOR FISS.-. CRESTING - CHARLES - BACHA
AND BLICK ... OUR WINNING TEAM
... THEY WILL KEEP YOU SAFE**

If the Defys managed to succeed and their candidates—Olga Yammo, Hani Singer, and Podes Diaz—won, maybe there was still time for a more peaceful evolution instead of a bloody revolution. It could set the course of humanity's survival in a whole new direction.

Dismantling Corporit rule would take hard work and dedication. And the worst thing that could happen?—revolution, confusion, and chaos all over the globe.

It might seem like an impossible task. The Corporits had been in power for thirty years and had ruled with an iron fist. Up against them were the Defys and no one really knew how many there were or if their message of democratic rule by the people had even taken root.

She looked up toward the sky.

Storm, are you there?

* * *

Storm had gone to see Laya earlier in the day. She seemed happy, skipping and laughing with the other children. Then she saw him—excited, she raced to him and hugged him around the waist.

"Where's Mommy?"

"She asked me to come and see you while she was away."

The little girl looked perplexed. "She didn't say she was going away."

Storm watched her eyes grow large with worry. He crouched down. "She'll be back soon, Laya."

Storm recognized one of the Aught children holding a teacher's hand. He looked frightened.

"Who is that boy?" Stormed nodded in the child's direction.

"He's brand new. His name is Daggo."

"He looks scared. Maybe he needs a friend like you." Storm watched Laya's face light up.

"I'll come back to see you tomorrow," Storm said. He gave her a hug; she kissed his cheek goodbye and skipped towards Daggo.

* * *

Asher Wind Storm merged into the swirling dust. He spun and climbed with the wind.

Higher and higher up in the sky.

Below he could see the spread of Caplac Domes. There were more and more of them every year, spilling over the land, covering most of the earth in the Noncorps sector and beyond.

His heart swelled with joy. He knew there were other domes far across the globe. His followers were spreading them everywhere.

Within them could be the seeds of humanity's tomorrows.

Maybe.

Maybe humans will someday come to respect the value of the Earth.

Understand the land should be as alive as the people who live on it.

Understand that without it there is no food, there is no air to breathe.

There is no life.

Tears filled his eyes and he descended.

Sadness was bringing him down.

Why can't they understand? Why can't I make them see?

He heard his mother's voice:

"All is chosen. They must find their way. Choose their own destiny."

Down.

Down.

Down.

Sanfrancorp's lights beamed out of the darkness.

He circled and circled.

Searching.

He searched for his love, searched for Zoe's life force.

Soon, like magic, it throbbed around him.

A warning choked off his joy.

She might not come back this time.

Chapter 47

EMORY DUTTON'S APARTMENT
Morning of CIC Hearing

Emory Dutton was frantic, his mind kept racing ahead to the proceedings in a few hours, alternating between the possible outcomes. One minute he envisioned a scenario of dismissal, the next, indictment. Now it was morning and he'd never closed his eyes.

Why hadn't he covered his tracks? Did he have to announce the accelerated stabilizer to every Medi-Prog chief? And in an open meeting? Why didn't he just slip it into the population through Pharmcorp, or make it available to the public without letting on he knew about its deadly use?

Those were the very questions his wife, Barbara, had asked when he told her about the hearing. She'd been merciless.

"Arrogant. Always need to be top dog," she said.

"I thought it was only fair to tell them," Dutton lamely fired back. "They're the ones who have to deal with the complications, the deaths."

"This is me, remember?" Barbara said. "What you really wanted was to flex your muscles, make sure they knew the kind of power you had over the whole medical system—over every single person."

She'd walked out of the room laughing. He was seeking some kind of solace, and instead he'd been crushed with the truth.

Dammit! It's the Quinns who're doing this to me. Payback for killing their miserable son.

It's all because of them and their foundation bringing up the charges. Everyone else would have complained—but in the end, simply gone along with his manipulation.

The Quinns have fought against any idea I've ever had. I've always said they have too much influence. Should have made it my number-one priority to get rid of them in the very beginning. I didn't try hard enough.

If only there were some way to get out of this hearing. But even his own Advocator had laughed at him, told him there was nothing he could do. Once summoned, there was no refusing to appear before the CIC.

Dutton had tried, but now he was cornered.

* * *

(30 hours earlier)

Emory Dutton picked up the telelink and punched in the private number of Adam Fiss. It rang awhile before the Chief Interrogator answered.

"What do you want, Emory? You woke me up and I'm not sleeping too well the way it is, with these damn elections coming up. You do know the day after tomorrow is the elections, don't you?"

"What I know is tomorrow is the day I've been subpoenaed to appear before the CIC. Fuck the election."

Dead silence.

"Are you there, Adam?"

"Since when did you think you could get away with talking to me like that?"

Adam Fiss's voice was soft, but there was a lethal undertone that Dutton hadn't heard tossed his way for years. Dutton was speechless.

"Now, was there something you wanted to ask me before I disconnect?" Adam said. "We shouldn't even be talking."

Dutton was really scared. His hands were shaking and he could barely hold onto the telelink.

"Do you think they have a solid case against me?"

"We won't know that until the hearing tomorrow," Adam said.

"Don't they have to submit their evidence to the court before a subpoena is issued?" Dutton could hear the tremor in his voice. It made him sound weak.

"No. This is strictly in the Advocator's ball park. He represents the Quinn Foundation and they are required to prove their case," Adam said.

"Nothing?" Dutton said.

"It's the only reason I took your call," Adam said. "I'm not going to get caught up in your mess. The only clue I have is the charge."

Dutton swallowed hard. "Crimes against humanity."

"That is the charge," Adam said sternly. "Now I suggest you try to get a good night's sleep. You're going to need it."

* * *

Emory Dutton had not entered his wife's bedroom in ten years. The last time he was there there she'd thrown him out for sleeping around with other women and humiliating her one time too many, not only privately, but with crowds of people watching and laughing.

She'd had nothing to do with him ever since.

He remembered the last time, he had threatened her for some little thing he couldn't even remember. "Do you want to end up in one of the harvesting tanks?"

She'd laughed in his face. "Go ahead. Do you think I haven't planted enough evidence to send you to hell? All my friends have the pieces of a puzzle that will put you into the criminal system. Maybe it's you who'll end up in one of the tanks."

Tonight he was desperate. When he edged into Barbara's shadowy room, the small bedside lamp gave out a weak glow.

231

He looked around and didn't recognize any of the furnishings. Besides a king-sized bed and a small dressing table, there was a love seat and a couple of small stuffed chairs. Many contemporary paintings, obviously done by the same artist, were hung on the walls. When he moved in closer, he saw his wife's name in the corner. She had painted all of them. When had she become an artist?

They were fascinating.

Her voice pierced the silence. "What do you want, Emory?"

"I wanted to talk to you, Barbara."

"Don't you think anything we had to say to each other has already been said?"

He moved closer to the bed. She turned over and looked up at him with steely eyes—not a hint of give.

"Can I come under the covers with you?" When there was no answer, he said, "Please."

"What do you want with this fat old, woman." Her voice was harsh, condemning. "Go to one of your other women ... why bother me now?"

"We used to love each other," he said. "Remember?"

Her voice lost its harshness. "That was a long time ago, Emory."

"Where did it all go wrong?" He tried to stand up tall but his legs were shaking and his heart was pounding hard against his chest.

"You stopped caring about me, our family. All you wanted was to be in charge ... be number one." She sat up. "We stopped mattering to you ... and then so did everyone else."

"But don't you remember ... everything was in such chaos? I only wanted to bring order."

Barbara's words were cruel, but her eyes were soft. "You've stepped on, crushed anyone or anything that stood in your way in your climb to the top." She looked away. "Emory, you've been responsible for the deaths of so many, I can't even begin to imagine what the total might be."

"I only wanted what was best for everybody."

She reached over and turned off the light. All that was left was the eerie light from the window. The room's deep shadows held terrors he hadn't thought of since he was a child.

Barbara moved to the other side of the bed.

Silently, he lifted the covers and edged in and found an old memory of comfort.

Bette Golden Lamb

Chapter 48

George Potek rode the elevator up to Emory Dutton's apartment. The CEO was expected to appear at the hearing before the CIC in less than an hour. Although there was no official protocol that required the CAPO commander take him in, Dutton had asked if he would accompany him.

At first Potek wanted laugh in his face. Why didn't he? He hated the man. Maybe it was only habit, or maybe stupidity, or rote, to do what he was told by Dutton.

Potek pressed on the door buzzer and to his surprise, the door was opened by Dutton's wife, Barbara.

"Come in, commander."

"Thank you, Mrs. Dutton."

She led the way to the kitchen where Dutton was drinking ice water, one glass after another.

Potek thought he'd be more elated at seeing Dutton so humbled, but somehow he felt a twinge of pity watching the CEO in his elegant suit, drinking his water with shaking hands.

"Good morning, sir."

"Well, what the fuck is so good about it?" Dutton's face had turned into a mask of anger and hatred. "Why do you always have to say some inane thing, Potek? You're as big a fool today as you've always been."

Stunned, Potek only nodded, wondering how just a moment ago he'd felt some kind of sympathy for the man. Potek looked at his watch. "I think it's time for us to leave, sir. We're going to be late."

"Did you get the limo, as I asked?"

"Sorry, I tried, but they wouldn't release it to me."

Potek had wanted to see this man go down. That's why he'd agreed to accompany him. Now he realized what a fool he was to say yes. He would just end up being his whipping boy ... again.

"Can't do a silly, simple, stupid, solitary task." Then Dutton laughed at what he thought was his own cleverness.

"Do you wish me to accompany you or not, sir?"

Dutton turned his back on the commander, walked up to his wife, who had witnessed the whole scene. His shoulders were thrown back and he seemed to have regained some of his usual stature. He was still facing her when he said, "What do you think, fool? Isn't that why I called you in the first place?"

Potek did not respond.

"Goodbye, Barbara. I'll see you later when all of this tiresome nonsense is finished."

She stood there, not uttering a word, but there was an air of sadness surrounding her silence.

Chapter 49

CIC Hearing

Chief Interrogator Adam Fiss sat on a raised podium, with Marinda Bacha and Cedra Cresting on his left and Gary Blick and Argaret Charles on his right. Their faces were solemn, but there was also an aura of nervous energy that Dutton always associated with the fear of the people summoned to his office.

Dutton stared back at the five of them from his table—his advocator sat next to him, fingers busy at his docuslate. The CEO turned to look at Becky and Tris Quinn, the leading officers of the Quinn Foundation. They sat at the other table with their advocator, who sat calmly looking up at the CIC members of the board.

Adam Fiss said: "Not a good way to begin these proceedings with a late arrival, Mr. Dutton."

Dutton's advocator jumped in. "We beg your pardon, sir. The streets are unusually congested with pedestrians."

"As you might imagine, I'm fully aware of that," Fiss said. "Yet all of us are here at the appointed hour."

"Yes, sir."

Dutton was having trouble following the formalities and the back and forth between his advocator and Adam Fiss. His mind was wandering, no matter how much he tried to concentrate. The proceeding seemed to go on a long time before he was asked a question by the Quinns' advocator. Dutton only snapped to attention when it was repeated in a sharp tone.

"Mr. Dutton, did you knowingly hire Pharmcorp, no, pardon me, it wasn't Pharmcorp, it was Drugcorp. Did you hire that company to create a tainted stabilizer?"

Dutton's advocator jumped up. "I object to that question. My client has maintained his innocence."

"Sit down," Fiss said coldly to the advocator. "Answer the question, Mr. Dutton."

"If you'll look at our corporate protocols, you can see I'm not involved with the ordering of materials," Dutton said. "I have never been in contact with any corporation for such an order."

Argaret Charles pointed a finger at Dutton. "Don't be obtuse, sir. Was the poisonous stabilizer ordered at your request, or not?" She nodded at Dutton's advocator. "Do not interfere. I want an answer to the question."

"No, I ordered a stabilizer for VMAS patients."

"Then, what did you think actually caused thousands across the globe to die?" Cedra Cresting asked.

"I never dreamed that Drugcorp had a tainted product." Dutton said. "I didn't find out about it until it was too late. Why should this rest at my doorstep? I'm as much an innocent victim as the ones who died."

Tris Quinn jumped up. "You're a miserable liar!"

Adam Fiss pounded on the table. "Sit down, Dr. Quinn. No more of that."

"May I say something, Chief?" the advocator said.

"Speak."

"The only reason the Quinn Foundation is pursuing these charges against my client, Emory Dutton, is to determine his part in the capture and killing of Drs. Becky and Tris Quinns'son."

"That has no relevance in this presentation today," Fiss said.

"Sir, I believe it does." The advocator shuffled the papers on the table.

"Your reasoning, sir." Fiss appeared miffed.

"My client doesn't deny his part in the death of Nathan Quinn. But that man and his cohort Seka Joraine were terrorists trying to destroy the Organ Harvesters complex. Mr. Dutton should be commended for his leadership in aborting a horrible crime."

"I certainly agree with CEO Dutton's advocator," Marinda Bacha said. "His quick thinking saved us from a medical disaster. All of our organ supplies could have been destroyed."

Dutton nodded at Marinda Bacha.

* * *

CAPO Commander George Potek sat at the back of the room. There were five chairs for visiting viewers of the proceedings. He was the only visitor.

I can't believe it; the bastard is going to get away with it.

Gary Blick spoke up at this time. "I have read some of your papers on population control, Mr. Dutton. I find your theories quite fascinating. The idea that anyone who is fatally ill should be immediately terminated, regardless of desire, is quite cogent. After all, it is for the greater good. Isn't that what the CIC is about?"

Dutton looked really pleased. He was starting to sit up taller and his shoulders were losing their slump.

"May I speak, Chief?"

"Speak."

Dutton stood. "We face a shrinking world. Life on the planet is threatened. If we are to survive we have to decrease the population. There are simply too many people on the planet."

"I assume you are to be one of the survivors?" Argaret Charles said. "Never mind. We all know the answer to that question."

George Potek liked that woman. He was glad he planned to vote for her and Cedra Crestin.

He could see how disappointed the Quinns were with the proceedings. If Dutton got off, Potek would seriously consider moving to the Noncorps. He'd heard about Asher Wind Storm and his Caplac Domes. Maybe if he could start all over again; he might find that there was something more than torturing people who were just trying to survive.

* * *

Dutton was losing the terror that had been a tight knot curled up in his bowels. Maybe this time he had outsmarted the Quinns and he would be found innocent.

"Bring in Dr. Andrew Potter," Chief Fiss asked a bailiff.

Potter!

Dutton hadn't worried about the medical chiefs. He knew they wouldn't dare testify against him. But he hadn't made the mistake of physically torturing any of them except the Chief of Robotics. Dutton had ordered his neural brain torture interrogation.

Andrew Potter walked in from a side door and sat down at the witness table.

"Thank you for coming today, doctor." Fiss said.

Potter nodded.

"I'll be frank, sir," Fiss said, "nothing we've heard here is strong enough to condemn Emory Dutton of crimes against humanity. In our society, there is no greater crime than one that deliberately destroys human life."

The Chief Interrogator then spoke directly to the Quinn Foundation advocator. "You may present your questions to the witness."

The advocator stood and walked over to Potter. "Thank you for coming today, sir."

Potter nodded.

"Did you attend a Medi-Prog meeting where CEO Emory Dutton stated he'd contaminated a stabilizing patch to end the lives of *anyone* with VMAS?"

"Yes. I was at that meeting."

"Are you sure you didn't misinterpret what the CEO stated?"

Andrew Potter looked directly into Dutton's eyes. "It was plainly stated. The vaccine would bring in everybody for inoculation and the adulterated stabilizer would eliminate everyone with VMAS."

"Is there anything else, sir?"

"It was to be given within a three-day window," Potter said.

"Why do you think it was presented that way, sir?"

"So the whole population would be vaccinated against VMAS. But infected people, although promised survival, would be terminated."

"Is there anything else, Doctor?"

"No."

When Andrew Potter left the room, Fiss said, "We will resume with our final judgment and dispensation tomorrow morning." He pointed a finger at Dutton.

"Please be on time, Mr. Dutton."

* * *

"Silence ruled as Potek and Dutton left the CIC building and walked to the van. Dutton was furious with the way the proceedings had ended. Frustrated, he wanted to strike the commander.

Was that a smug look on his face? After all I've done for the bastard.

Once inside the van, Dutton shouted, "Get me out of here!"

"Yes, sir."

"Damn it, they're trying to railroad me."

"Sorry, sir?"

"I have one more year in office and they'll see what happens when they need my help." Dutton turned to Potek. "Right now that Marinda Bacha needs a new kidney. She'd better do the right thing" He waved a hand in the air. "Or puff, gone."

"Yes, sir."

"She'll just have to hop along with the one failing kidney she was born with. Bitch."

"Yes, sir."

"And Adam Fiss? We all know about his liver ... the drinking bastard. What young, beautiful bitch's liver is going to save his life without me?"

Dutton looked out the window. "Did I ask to go home, you idiot? Take me to my office. Once there, Dutton got out of the van and slammed the door with all the strength he had.

* * *

Astrid, get your ass into my office," Dutton said. "And I mean right now."

"Yes, Mr. Dutton." She looked away, as every person he saw did, but she was quick to follow him into his office.

She'll be sorry ... they'll all be sorry.

"Get me Adam Fiss on the telelink and I don't want any excuses. Get him!"

Dutton couldn't sit. He walked to his window and stared out across at the city streets.

You people are ants. A bunch of goddam insects. Nothings.

When he turned, Astrid was back again at the doorway. "They won't put me through."

"Who are they?"

"His office staff."

"Get out of here, you featherhead. That's what I get for using a wiggly ass instead of someone with brains."

Dutton sat down at his desk. Adrenalin coursed through every part of him. He grabbed his private telelink from his bottom drawer and hit Fiss's private line.

It rang and rang. Dutton waited until Adam finally picked up.

There were no preliminaries. "I told you I can't speak to you during this hearing. It's not legal."

"It's not legal, huh?" Dutton said. "Well, there's a lot you do that's not legal—"

"Listen, Emory. I can't do anything until after the election."

"You know, it's strange how all the biggest hypocrites in the world are the ones who blow their livers drinking. Some of them are your best friends. They're the biggest customer group I

242

have for my little Organ Harvesters health plan." Dutton laughed into the phone.

"Are you threatening me?" Adam said.

"Damn right I am," Dutton said. "Do this right or you better get used to the color yellow for the short time you'll have without a functioning liver."

"Look, Emory, I'm trying. But hell, you only have a year left in office anyway," the chief interrogator said. "Why don't you just run?"

"Run! I'm not running anywhere. Just remember, if I go down, you go down, too."

Bette Golden Lamb

Chapter 50

CORPORIT ELECTIONS DAY

Bacha Residence

Jin barely heard Melik when he came home in the early morning hours. She wakened when his hands raked over her body ... fingering, poking, violating. He yanked her onto her back, tore off her nightgown while the stink of sour booze blew across her face. Then he climbed on top of her.

"Leave me alone!" she screamed. "Leave me alone!"

"You'll do what I say, when I tell you, bitch."

"I hate you!" she yelled, scratching his arms, his face. "Get off of me."

He pried her legs apart and forced his way inside and hammered her while she pounded his chest. Nothing stopped him until he was finished.

She spit in his face. "Rapist pig!"

Spent, he'd passed out on top of her, mouth open, his drool running down her cheek. When she shoved him aside, he rolled to the floor—out cold; he began to snore.

She fled from the bed, dressed, and ran from their apartment.

* * *

Andrew was sound asleep when the doorman called on his telelink. He listened, then replied, "Yes."

When the elevator door snapped open, Jin stood looking up at him. Her face was blanched white and her eyes were like black marbles flung in the snow.

He opened his arms and gathered her to him, carried her to the bed, carefully undressed her and wrapped them together in the warm blankets. He murmured soothing tones. "Shhhhh. Everything will be all right."

She sobbed into his shoulder. "Andrew ... oh my god ... he hurt me ... hurt me so ... it was so awful."

Andrew's colleagues always accused him of being as cold hearted and unemotional as his robotic creations. But all he wanted was to take a dull knife and cut off Melik's balls.

"Forgive me ... I'm so sorry ... I know we weren't supposed to see each other ... but there was nowhere else I could go and feel safe. I had to be with you."

"Don't think about it." He clutched her tighter. "I'm glad you're here with me."

They fell asleep tight in each other's arms.

* * *

The light streamed in the window. Andrew and Jin awakened at almost the same instant.

Jin looked at Andrew. His dark skin was smooth, his soft eyes searched hers. "Why didn't I meet you years ago instead of Melik?"

He gently trailed a finger down her cheek. "None of that matters anymore. We've finally found each other." He drew her into a kiss that she never wanted to end.

When they pulled apart, she whispered, "I love you, Andrew, and I wish we could stay here all day. But I have to go to the office." She sat up. "Today is the day and if I don't help push the slate to beat the incumbents ... well, it will be the same old, same old CIC. I have to give Yammo, Singer, and Diaz every chance to win."

"It's true. We need you," Andrew, whispered back, hoping to defeat any listening devices. "But I can't ask you to risk your life anymore. It's much too dangerous." He reached out, clasped her to him, squeezed her as though he would never let her go.

"If there's to be a future ... any hope at all for us, I have to do what I can." She moved from his arms and walked into the bathroom to get ready.

After a long shower, she picked up her clothes, which were fairly presentable although she made a face at them, and dressed. They would have to do because she was never going back to the apartment she shared with Melik.

Andrew, already dressed, was straightening the bed. "Today is the last day the Defys will have to get their message out." He looked away. "I wish I was the one to do what you have to do ... but you're it. You're the only one left in News-Div that can help us win."

"I know."

"We've been secretly pushing our message for six years—I think the people are behind us. If we can't unseat the present CIC, the Corporit system will prevail. Can we afford to wait six more years? I doubt it."

"I think you should know, Marinda Bacha has insisted I get her name out there. She's using our relationship, dangling it from a string. She'll tell Melik and the Bacha family about us if I don't blast her name out on the news strips—she's determined to win, no matter how the other incumbents do."

"Like brother, like sister."

* * *

"I have to leave," Jin said. Andrew looked at her and there was only sadness in his eyes.

"Please don't go." He held onto her arm as though that could keep her from leaving. "I know I was the one that asked you to do this, but if they catch you ... Jin, I can't bear the thought of losing you."

"I have to do something worthwhile, Andrew, something that will make a difference. Since I married Melik five years ago, I've been playing a role, walking without seeing anything around me."

"All the suffering the Corporits have caused while I fast-forwarded to avoid seeing any of those realities She moved into his arms and kissed him. "If I'd only cared enough to look at what our life had become."

"Don't be so hard on yourself." Andrew said. "You're not the enemy."

"My Aunt Becky and Uncle Tris used to poke me about keeping my head in the sand. My comeback: I'm a journalist, how much more into the fray can you get than that?"

"Well, that family of yours never lets up," he said, laughing. "But without them, and people like them ... well, I know things would be even worse."

"But, Andrew, don't you see? I was kidding myself. When you're told what to write by the people in charge, that's not what a journalist is supposed to do. We're supposed to tell the truth, no matter what."

"We all do the best we can," Andrew said, kissing her cheek. "Ethan Taylor did the right thing and looked what happened to him."

"At least he tried his best. And Andrew, you've done the best you can, too. Your neck is on the line. That hasn't stopped you. And your friend Zoe? She was safe ... she left her daughter and a new life ... to do the right thing. What have I done? I only married into a wealthy Corporit family that perpetuates all that's wrong with this crushing system."

"There was no way you could have known what the Organ Harvesters were really about." Andrew sat up. "Dutton and all of the Corporits are on an island of immortality that floats on the backs of the rest of us. They made sure you didn't know."

"But I *do* know now, and I won't go back just because it's safe."

They suddenly reached out and wrapped their arms around each other. She kissed every part of his face, desperate to take in all of him.

Then, she was gone.

* * *

News-Div Offices

Jin was jumpy. She placed two fingers on the entrance identification lock at the News-Corp building and walked through darkened corridors into the News-Div section. There, she keyed in her pass code to slip inside.

Even though it was an election day, the offices of News-Div were dark. No one had come into work early. Why bother when yesterday they were all given the stories they each would submit—told exactly how to write them. Even the streaming news strips had been preprogrammed.

She'd never been inside when there was no one else around. It was pretty creepy. She kept waiting for someone to jump out and grab her.

Seated at her desk, Jin looked out the window, watched the bright news strips circulate around every building in sight. They all said the same thing. The same information they'd been running the whole pre-election month: Pushing the incumbent candidates, making sure they burned into every voter's brain. That along with bashing the Noncorp and Aught terrorists that didn't exist, but were coming to kill them.

She got comfortable in her seat close to the window and started up—she was online almost instantly. She began to sabotage the communication system.

People going to work in an hour would see the news strips and hear the Defys' preprogrammed blasts around the city. When it was all keyed in, she would jam all the communication mechanisms in the News-Div's office, leaving the strip she created continuing to flash across the buildings. They would never have the system back and functioning until late today, after the polls were closed.

Her knees turned to water. She hesitated and began to shake all over.

249

What am I doing? Why am I doing this?

Then she took a deep breath, cinched in her gut. Today she was going to be a real journalist. She would tell the truth: they'd been living under a system that had put technological advancements ahead of human rights and protection of the environment. Today, everyone would know it was time for change. They would know each individual could make a difference. No matter what happened to her, people needed to know their vote could change everything.

Chapter 51

CIC HEARING
Dutton's Final Appearance

The speakers on the top of the buildings were all blasting continuously. Dutton's ears were tingling with the sound as they walked to the unmarked cruiser.

VOTE FOR YAMMO.-. SINGER.-.DIAZ ... THE CANDIDATES WE NEED FOR CHANGE ... JOIN THE DEFYS TODAY ... WE WILL BRING BACK DEMOCRACY

The news strips circled around and around every structure:

The Corporate-Government Coalition Has Brought A Global Corporit Dictatorship ... Its Legacy? ... Escalating Climate Change ... Limited Food Supplies ... Clean Air Only For The Elite

* * * Special News Bulletin * * *
Medical Programmer CEO Emory Dutton Appears Again Before CIC - Charged With Crimes Against Humanity ... Is He Guilty?

People in the streets were pointing to the news strips and they were smiling.

"Get me out of here, Potek."

"Yes, sir."

"Sir, sir, sir. Yes, sir, no sir. Can't you ever come up with anything else. Dammit, that noise is driving me crazy."

"Yes, sir."

Potek drove the cruiser but it was difficult to maneuver through the crowds that had amassed everywhere. There were even clots of people dancing in the streets, all of them pointing up to the tops of the buildings.

"Isn't Morgenthau still in charge at News-Corp?" Dutton shouted, trying to hear his own voice. "What kind of headlines are those? Terrorists must have gotten to them."

"No, sir. There's been no terrorist activity in Sanfrancorp."

"Oh, I forgot what great protectors you and your CAPOs are." Dutton's voice dripped sarcasm. "I'll bet there's not one Defy in the whole city because of your fine efforts. Their existence is just a nasty rumor."

Potek was silent.

"Nothing to say? You're a poor excuse for a commander. Or have I said that before?" Dutton was screaming at Potek now. "You can kiss that cushy job of yours goodbye. There's plenty more little companies ready to take on the big boys. You can just slip into a well-deserved obscurity."

CEO Emory Dutton Faces CIC ... Accused Of Crimes Against Humanity

Dutton wanted to put his fist through the van's glass window. His heart was racing and his head was throbbing with a migraine. He couldn't remember the last time he was this angry.

"Is this what it comes down to in the end?" Dutton said. "Those fools are going to tell the corporations how to run things."

People in the streets continued to point to the news strips and they were smiling.

"We're here, sir."

Bette Golden Lamb

Chapter 52

NEWS-DIV

Reporters, PR, media people, all from the various divisions in News-Corp were crowding into the News-Div office. Everyone was buzzing with excitement.

Jin had expected to take a verbal beating over what she'd done. But once one of the senior staff members admitted he was a Defy, most of the others began to jumping in with the same admission. They all agreed this election was the moment they'd been waiting for to take a stand. Now or never! They began hammering Jin with questions:

"When did you get to be such a gutsy thing?"

"Do you think any of the new candidates will get in?"

"God, I hope so. "

"Can't let the Corporits have another six years."

"Hell, I'd have been scared to death."

"When did you grow a pair, Jin?"

Everything was coming at her at once. It was too much. She looked at them and her mind went blank, then she burst into tears. The room went silent.

Alex Becker, one of their top senior reporters, broke through the people surrounding her, placed a hand on her shoulder. "Most of us have been here a long time ... certainly many more years than you. Some even saw the world before the Corporits. We haven't liked these changes, but none of us did anything about it until now."

Jin looked up at the older man who had been the most supportive in her efforts to learn the profession. She smiled at him.

"You," Becker continued, "nothing more than a cub reporter, have led the way." He bent over and kissed her cheek. "Thanks, Jin."

Everyone in the room started clapping and hooting.

Sudden, strident voices pierced the cheering. Men pushed through the crowd. "Step aside! Step aside!"

Six private security guards shoved people out of their way—cutting a path for Jin's husband, Melik, who strutted up to her. Without a word, he slapped her face so hard she almost fell out of the chair. Needle points of pain stabbed at her face, but she forced herself to sit up tall and glare at him.

"What the hell do you think you're doing?" Becker said, trying to shoulder one of the guards out of the way. The crowd started elbowing and pushing.

Another reporter yelled, "Are you nuts?"

Melik nodded and the guard grabbed Alex Becker by the arm, yanked him around, then tasered him until he fell over in a heap, grasping for air.

"We have plenty of the same for anyone of you who'd like it ... come on, step right up," Melik said, looking around.

"Please don't." Jin blurted to the crowd. "It'll only make things worse."

Melik laughed. He grabbed Jin's arm and yanked her out of the chair.

Chapter 53

ROBOTICS FACILITY

Andrew Potter was shocked to learn that none of the other department chiefs were willing to testify as he had, and they'd all been asked. Dutton would have gotten off if Andrew hadn't stepped up. Although Dutton's conviction wasn't a sure thing, at least the CIC knew the truth.

Would they dare to let the Emory Dutton off on an election day?

To think I'd been delighted when they moved the CIC world headquarters to Sanfrancorp from New York City. Ironically, at the same site where the former United Nations first met.

Maybe it would have been better if I didn't have to deal with them up close and personal.

He smiled at his assistant, the spy, and said, "I'll be in a meeting discussing a new robotic neural technique ... gone a little over an hour."

"Who's the meeting with?" she asked.

"Why do you want to know?" He bent over her desk.

I've got to admit those pheromones are pretty damn enticing.

"Oh, just curious."

"Just another robotics brain surgeon."

"You sure do have a lot of new techniques," she leaned over until they were almost touching."

He looked her right in the eye, no smile this time. "That's why they call me a genius. See you later."

Andrew didn't have to have eyes in the back of his head to know she would pick up her telelink and report to someone.

* * *

POTEK'S CAPO OFFICE

Potek received the call from Andrew Potter's assistant. "Thank you for your information."

There was little doubt that the Chief of Robotics was up to something, and had been for a long time. But Potek sat back in his chair and ignored the call just as he had a number of calls about the Quinns and their underground hospital meetings. And he still hadn't reported to Dutton the fact that Becky Quinn made an unauthorized visit to the Organ Harvesters complex a couple of nights ago.

He'd been a CAPO commander much too long and he was burned out, disgusted with the whole business—he was ready to try something else. Something where he'd never have to see Dutton, or people like him, again.

* * *

CORPORIT UNIDENTIFIED WAREHOUSE

Once Andrew Potter left his office, he picked up the pace and hurried to the ambulated walkway. The briefcase he'd removed from a rental locker was getting heavy.

He took precautions, checked to see if anyone was following him.

It was strange—he'd been followed since the time he'd been picked up by the CAPOs and taken to Dutton for interrogation. Every single day.

Today there was no one.

He jumped off at a secluded part of the city, walked a block to an isolated warehouse surrounded by a twelve-foot electrified fence. There was a small gate where authorized people could enter.

C, from his Defy cell, was there waiting for him. He carried a case like Andrew's.

"Let's get to it, Carl."

No matter what happened after today, Andrew was excited. The Defys had waited for this day for six long years.

Both of them opened their briefcases—foot pedals fell to the ground from inside each of their cases.

Entry required two separate, matched identification devices. They placed their fingers on the gate ID plates, tapped the foot pedals, which sent signals obliterating a record of their unauthorized visit. The gate sprang open.

Two robot guards approached Carl and Andrew.

"May I help you?" They both spoke at the same time. One to Andrew, one to Carl.

"Fifteen minute down time, commencing now!" Andrew said. Both robots instantly became inactive.

"When did you implant voice recognition? I didn't think that was part of their programming," Carl said as they walked to the entry to the warehouse.

Andrew laughed. "It's not, except for my voice. I stuck it in under the wire."

"Why only fifteen minutes? You told me it would probably take us at least twenty minutes to fix this," Carl said, opening the door.

"The CAPOs will be here in twenty minutes, no matter what command I give." Andrew clapped Carl on the shoulder. "I can only get away with so much when it comes to security."

Carl gave him a nervous smile. "Well, let's move it."

"How do like this mother ship?" Andrew said, waving at the huge spread of computers inside the warehouse.

"So this is where all the votes come in and are tallied?" Carl tried to speak calmly, but was obviously jumpy and ready to run at any time.

"This is it," Andrew said, checking his watch. He walked up to an inconspicuous side panel and tapped in a code. A large door slid open. "You can plug into that aperture ... I'll plug into mine."

"Just tell me what to do. I'm a brain surgeon, not a computer nerd."

"When I say go, enter the program in your case—it will initiate a virus that will wipe out any outside Corporit entries meant to tamper with the machine in any way. Only the votes that are cast will be tallied later today."

Andrew watched Carl download the program. "Okay," Andrew said. He downloaded his program with rapid finger movements. "I've shut down the existing outside connections that are already housed inside the tally program. Today we're going to have a real election."

"A real election?" Carl said.

"Every vote will be untampered with and counted . The people will get exactly the kind of representation they vote for."

* * *

Andrew and Carl left the warehouse in exactly fourteen minutes, zipping up their briefcases as they ran for the entry gate. Carl slipped and fell. Andrew grabbed his briefcase as he got back up.

"Run!"

They ran full out, slipping and sliding on the gravelly surface. Andrew's watch beeped fifteen minutes exactly when they closed the entry gate behind them.

The inactive robots began walking back and forth around the perimeter close to the gate, as though they suspected someone entering.

"We can't be seen together. You go ahead of me," Andrew said. "Run until you get to ambulated walkway. The CAPOs will be here any minute."

Carl took off.

Andrew wasn't too far behind. He had almost reached the entrance of the walkway when he heard the CAPOs' sirens in the distance.

Four hovervans pulled up to the gate they'd just run from. They were tapping in their identification when Andrew turned away and ran to step on the moving belt.

Chapter 54

It seemed like Jin had been in the security van forever. They'd blindfolded her and it wasn't until they were stopped and parked that Melik pulled her from the vehicle and snatched off the cloth covering her eyes.

She tried to look around but he yanked her arm, dragging her into a large warehouse. The four security guards followed them. It was dimly lit, dusty, and smelled of old sweat. Without a word, Melik pushed her into a straightback chair with arm rests. He nodded at the men and they backed off.

His black, curly hair was wet with sweat and his eyes were like gray stone.

"Did I not make myself perfectly clear?"

Jin had been filled with fear when he'd taken her from the News-Div offices and throughout the ride to this miserable warehouse. It was obviously at the edge of the city. She was resigned to anything that might happen to her. She'd had no illusions about surviving her act of sabotage.

"Clear about what?" she finally said.

He walked up to her, bent over and looked her in the eyes before he slapped her face. "You little bitch. You know exactly what."

"What I do know, Melik ... you raped me." Her face burned where he'd slapped her. "You are nothing but a miserable excuse for a man."

That immediately earned her another slap, this time on the other cheek. "Don't play games with me. I promised my sister you would get her name out in the news strips ... with a positive hit of information. Anything to make it easier for her to regain her seat on the CIC."

"What you promise Marinda is between you and her. I have nothing to do with it."

Melik stepped away from her. "Now I look like an inept, damn fool."

Jin laughed, couldn't stop herself, "I don't think I'll touch that one."

"It would be so easy to finish you off after those news reports you dumped out to the public," Melik said, his face a scarlet red. "In fact, lots of people are going to want a piece of you."

"You're so into ownership you seem to think I belong to you. What you forget ... I'm a Quinn," she said. "Whatever you do to me will get you into real trouble."

"And you overrate your family's influence."

Jin smiled. "I think we both know that's a lie."

He sounded like a petulant little boy. "Why couldn't you just give Marinda a little something ... for me?"

"Because your sister is as self-centered as you are and she doesn't deserve to be reelected."

Melik turned away but when he faced her again, his voice was icy cold. "You better hope she wins ... and you're going to sit right here until we find out."

* * *

The Quinns' Apartment

Tris didn't know what to say to his brother Jacob. Jin's father was barely holding it together as the three of them sat in Becky and Tris's living room. They had to do something, but Tris wasn't sure what.

"You say they grabbed her at the office?" Becky said, tears running down her cheeks.

"Alex Becker is a close friend and colleague of Jin's. He called me as soon as they took her away," Tris said.

Tris watched Jin's father sink lower and lower into his chair. "I told her not to marry that self-centered, idiot Melik. She wouldn't even talk to me about it, but she never had much faith in herself. I think she was afraid she'd never get married."

"You really think so?" Becky said. "I think she was in love with him at one point.

"I've never been able to make rhyme or reason out of why people do anything. Why should this be any different?"

"But the Bacha family," Jacob said. "The whole bunch are nothing more than Corporit pirates."

"I'll bet Marinda was furious with the newscasts," Becky said, her face flushing. "Somehow we've got to get Jin away from Melik."

Jacob bowed his head. "I can't find her. I've checked everywhere."

* * *

The thing that had sparked Zoe's journey back to Sanfrancorp was the death of the Aught woman who had come to the domes to save herself. She remembered helping Godan and his followers. She hoped they all went to the domes, where they could survive with dignity and hope.

But in Sanfrancorp, even in her sleep, there was never any rest for Zoe. It was hard to stop thinking about the things she'd done since leaving Storm.

In endless nightmares, everyone returned again to remind her of her journey: The sick and dying Aughts and their death-filled encampment; her drowning with a suffering child in a holding tank in the Organ Harvesters, its skeletal arms clutching at her, squeezing her closer and closer in a death grip. Even dying, she could hear the spider drones and their click-click-click-click. She shivered, covered her ears; the armies of drones clattered relentlessly in her brain. She was always running—running from the Corporits, from CAPOS, from Dutton, from the Organ Harvesters.

The gory nightmares awakened her. She was soaked in cold sweat, shaking and terrified. She'd come to help Andrew and the Defys, done the best she could. Her friend now had the information he needed, but Zoe was exhausted. It was time for her to leave, to gather her strength for the trip back to Storm and Laya, to return to her future home.

Thinking about her daughter made her happy. Her little girl had been through hell, and part of it was Zoe's fault. It was time to leave and be with her.

A tapping at the door tore her away from her thoughts. At first, she resisted answering, but when the knocking persisted, she picked up a knife from the kitchen table and tucked it into a pocket.

"Yes?" she said to the closed door.

"Zoe, it's Tris." He spoke so softly, it took a moment for the name to connect. She opened the door and he rushed inside.

"Tris, what are you doing here? This is not safe for either of us."

"I know, but I had to come. Melik has grabbed Jin." He sat down in the seat. "He came right to News-Div with his own security guards and took her away. Jacob is going crazy ... we all are."

Her heart started racing, for a moment she couldn't breathe. "I've got to get to Andrew; he's the only one who can help us." Zoe paced around the room. She felt caged and useless. "The longer Jin's gone the more danger she's in."

* * *

Zoe had to travel through the transpod to get to Andrew's apartment. The raucous noise from the speakers on the buildings was overwhelming, but it did distract people from looking at her.

VOTE FOR YAMMO - SINGER - DIAZ ... THE CANDIDATES WE NEED FOR CHANGE ... JOIN THE DEFYS TODAY ... WE WILL BRING BACK DEMOCRACY

Streaming news panels on every building circled around and around:

THE CORPORIT-GOVERNMENT COALITION HAS CREATED A GLOBAL DICTATORSHIP ... IT'S LEGACY? ... ESCALATING CLIMATE CHANGE ... LIMITED FOOD SUPPLIES ... AND CLEAN AIR ONLY FOR THE ELITE

There was real excitement. Strangers were talking to each other and for the first time in years, Zoe could see optimism on people's faces everywhere she went.

Jin had done it! She'd helped to get the message out to everyone.

Andrew was leaving his apartment building when Zoe caught up to him. She ran and took hold of his arm. "I'm so glad I caught you."

He was startled, but he drew Zoe next to him and kept them moving. "You shouldn't have come. It's way too dangerous."

"I had to come. Your telelink was shut down."

"I didn't want to talk to anyone ... at least for—"

Zoe squeezed his arm. "You need to know, Melik kidnapped Jin right out of the News-Div office."

"What?" Andrew's eyes widened and his skin turned a ghastly gray.

"He'll kill her," Zoe said. "Tris Quinn told me all about the Bachas—huge Dutton fans."

"Dutton is a son of a bitch! He's been the cause of all of this. At least with some luck the CIC will do the right thing and find that bastard guilty as charged."

Zoe watched Andrew's shoulders droop, his face sag with worry. She took his hand, then hugged him. "Let's see what we can do for Jin."

"I've lost her, Zoe. Oh my god, it's all my fault. I've lost her."

Bette Golden Lamb

Chapter 55

Outside Sanfrancorp's Dome

The ambulated walkway carried them under the protective dome to the last stop on the mass transit line. Zoe was on stimulants, trying to keep up her energy, but her muscles were still sluggish.

"It's somewhere around here, somewhere in this deserted district outside of the city," Andrew said. "When we arrived, I was in a vehicle with my eyes covered. I didn't get enough of a glimpse to really identify the warehouse. But it's the only one of the Bachas' facilities listed outside of the dome-covered protected zone—the map says it should be here."

"But how can you be so sure?" Zoe said. "You've said their corporation owns fifty of them."

"All the rest are in the city limits. Look, the air in the warehouse where Melik interrogated me was contaminated. It wasn't hard to tell that there were no air scrubbers operating to make it safe. It was hard to breathe."

"But you were very upset after being attacked and kidnapped. You could be wrong."

"No. It was just outside of the city protective dome. I saw where the enclosure ended on my way back to the ambulated walkway."

It was starting to get dark and they'd spent a long time getting outside of Sanfrancorp's city limits. Zoe knew if they didn't soon locate the spot where Melik had taken Jin, it might be too late.

"She's probably safe until the election results are in," Andrew said, obviously trying to reassure himself.

Zoe looked at her watch. "Andrew that's in only 45 minutes."

"This is it!" Andrew pointed to a block building that looked rundown and there were no vehicles or people or signs of activity around it. "This is where Bacha took me when he kidnapped me."

Zoe was having trouble breathing. Without the city's protective dome, breathing in the open air was putting them both at risk for pulmonary shutdown.

"You're sure this is the place?"

"I gave up being sure about anything a long time ago," he said.

The light was fading fast as they walked on the gravelly surface towards a side door. Andrew pulled a gun from his back waistband.

"Are you going to use that?" she asked.

"If I have to, you bet I will."

Zoe hated the noise their steps were making, but there was no way around it. Gravel was noisy and even though it looked deserted, there could still be people inside holding Jin prisoner.

He reached for the broken door handle, looked at Zoe. She nodded and they burst into a huge, empty warehouse with a lone empty seat in the middle.

Andrew screamed out, "Son-of-a-bitch!"

* * *

Melik shoved Jin, gave her a couple of hard-hitting body punches the minute they walked into their apartment. Then he spoke to the security guards, dismissing them. "If I can't handle this little thing, then I'm the one who deserves to be beaten."

The men laughed as they walked out.

Jin's hands were tied behind her back and no matter how much she struggled, she couldn't break loose. He pushed her onto the couch in the living room.

"In twenty minutes we'll know the election results. You'd better hope for your sake that Marinda wins back her seat." He

270

pointed a finger at her. "I should have waited in that warehouse, but I don't like breathing air I can see. Why should I suffer with you, you miserable bitch?"

The telelink buzzed. Melik answered right away when he saw who was calling. He put it on speaker, glared at Jin.

"Hi, sis. Anything new?"

"New? No, there's nothing new. But I'm really pissed at you. I can't believe you can't control your own wife. Couldn't get her to put in a plug for her sister-in-law." Marinda's voice boomed across the room. "I told you not to marry her, no matter what father said."

"I know," he said. "You're right. She screwed us over."

"Well, you know what to do."

"Yeah, I know," Melik said. "But didn't you want her stashed until the final election results?"

"What difference does it make?" Marinda started bawling. "Damn, I need that win."

"So what," he said. "Forget it! You've got plenty of money. You don't really *need* that seat."

"Money?" Her voice was loud and angry. "Do you think that's what being on the CIC is about?"

Melik shot Jin a nasty leer. "I'm sorry. I know it's important to you. I only meant you'll be all right if it doesn't work out."

"You listen to me and let me make this clear. You will kill her. K-I-L-L H-E-R. That's always been *my* plan and you stick to it, no matter what." There was a long pause. "And make sure I get her kidneys because I need them. Do you understand?"

"Yeah, Marinda. I do."

"Good. Then I forgive you."

She disconnected.

Melik tossed the telelink away and walked up to the couch. He grabbed Jin's face by the chin and yanked it back and forth.

"You've never been pretty and those bruises aren't making you any better looking."

"Why did you marry me?" she said through her blood-caked mouth.

"Smart woman? A journalist? And you still haven't figured that out?" He pulled out a gutting knife from his back pocket.

Although she said nothing, she was shaking.

"My father told me to marry you. When he says jump, I jump."

"But why?" she said, her words blurring.

"You're a Quinn, aren't you? Dad and Dutton cooked up the whole scheme. They wanted a Quinn connection."

"So, you never loved me?" Goose bumps erupted all over when he cut his way through her blouse and bra. Then with a fast slash, he sliced though her underwear and pants. They split apart, clean and neat—like the belly of a fish.

"Loved you? The point was to make you love *me*. Besides, you were good in bed. That was my consolation prize."

"Well, I did love you until I saw what you were really like." She laughed at him. "By the way, how's that Quinn-Bacha alliance working out for you?"

"You figure it out. You're lying here with your hands tied because you fucked over my sister." He leaned over her face. "Didn't you, bitch?" He moved down and bit hard into her breast until she screamed.

"Stop!"

She tried to writhe from side to side, but he held her flat by grabbing her around the neck. He took the point of the knife and cut a long stripe from her breast bone to her navel. Blood welled up chasing the knife.

"Leave me alone, Melik. Please! Please! Please!"

He pulled his belt off, unzipped his fly and let himself flop out. Even with her hands tied, she fought him. But he drew her legs up and apart, thrust himself inside of her.

"One more time, baby. This is what you're good for. The only thing you're good for. This is why I haven't bashed your head in for the past five years."

Chapter 56

Dutton At Home

Dutton sat in his living room drinking, his best Scotch, watching the teleview. He occupied one end of the sofa, his wife, the other end.

"Thank you, Barbara. It was kind of you to sit with me."

She was silent.

An announcer stood next to a tally machine that was hooked into the main computers at an undisclosed location. The numbers were changing every few minutes next to the names of the nine candidates running for the five available seats."

"As you all know, this is the first election.
in six years for the important five seats on the
Corporit International Council.

The incumbents are: Chief Interrogator Adam Fiss,
 Cedra Cresting, Marinda Bacha, Gary Blick, Argaret Charles.

The four challengers are: Olga Yammo, Hani Singer,
Mitchell Payette, Podes Diaz."

Dutton broke out into a cold sweat and his heart tore at his chest. If Fiss was reelected he had a chance, but only if the four other members were true Corporits. Change was not something that would benefit him.

"Come on, come on." He took in another gulp of Scotch, tapped his feet and downed the liquor as though it were water. His hot skin felt like it would split open at any moment.

Barbara finally spoke. "Calm down, Emory. This is not doing you any good. The tally will be ready when it's ready."

"What the fuck do you know or care? It's not your life."

There was a long beat of silence. "You threw me away," she said, "kept me out of your life a long time ago. Sleeping with other women, keeping mistresses—I could go on and on." She stood. "Crudely put, I don't give a fuck ... and that's only the second time I've ever used that word in my life."

"Yeah, yeah, when was the first time?" He sneered at her. "You'd think I'd remember that, if I cared."

"I don't expect you to remember the first and last time you ever had an opportunity to strike me."

As she left the room, she threw back over her shoulder, "I wish you no harm, Emory, but if it means you get what you deserve ... well, so be it."

"Who cares what you think, you old hag."

"Fellow Corporits, we now have the final vote tally."

Dutton watched the numbers scroll across the screen.

"Our CIC for the next six years: Chief Interrogator, Adam Fiss has retained his seat."

He was up from the sofa, screaming, "There you go, Adam. Thank God!"

The announcer continued:

Cedra Cresting: Elected, Marinda Bacha: Not elected.
Gary Blick, Not elected, Argaret Charles: Elected.
Olga Yammo: Not elected, Hani Singer: Elected.
Mitchell Payette: Not Elected, Podes Diaz: Elected.

So as you can see, these are your newly elected CIC members:

Adam Fiss: Incumbent, Cedra Cresting: Incumbent.
Argaret Charles: Incumbent, Hani Singer: New Member.
Podes Diaz: New Member.

Dutton was up and circling the room. He felt as though his chest would explode.

"Ungrateful bastards. What the hell do the common people know? All they do is multiply ... grow, grow, and grow in a shrinking world. It's those damn Defys. They've ruined everything."

* * *

Jin screamed at Melik as he threw her to his van. "Where are you taking me?"

Melik looked at his wife. Her face was a mass of bruises and the inside of the robe he'd thrown on her was covered in blood, oozing from where he'd sliced her.

Should have gone deeper, gutted her, slit her all the way.

Couldn't take a chance on the fuckin' CAPOs crawling down my throat. And Marinda would freak.

Jin started screaming—the sound filled the van. He flung an arm out across her face—felt her nose crack under the blow. "Shut up!"

* * *

"Tris, it's me, Andrew. I've got Zoe Hidalga with me. We're going to get Jin."

"They're going to kill her, I know it. All because she's a Quinn. Those bastards. It wasn't bad enough losing a son, now they're going to kill my niece."

"We don't have time, Tris. We have to move on this. Listen, I need wheels. Can you get me a vehicle of some kind?"

"We never use it, but Becky has a van."

"I need it now." Andrew knew he was shouting, but he couldn't stop himself.

"Where are you?" Tris asked in a whisper.

"We're at Jin and Melik's apartment."

"We'll be there in fifteen minutes."

Andrew swallowed hard against the bile crawling up his throat. "Try to make it sooner."

Chapter 57

CIC CONFERENCE ROOM

Adam Fiss looked at the other members of the CIC. Now that the election was finished and tallied, he realized this body of members would only have one last decision to make.

Marinda Bacha looked as though she was taking her loss very hard. Gary Blick was probably just as glad to finally be done with an obligation that seemed to always conflict with his golfing dates.

C.C. and Argaret Charles were nothing but smiles.

Adam had mixed feelings. He had hoped things would stay the same, but this new CIC panel would definitely change things. He had a very strong hunch life was going to be drastically altered, but he wasn't sure exactly how.

"Well, it's getting very late and it's time we concluded our arguments and finalized our decision on the accusation brought forth by the Quinn Foundation re CEO Emory Dutton and crimes against humanity."

Marinda's face was bright red as she blurted, "What crimes? He made a unilateral decision to get rid of a lot of sick people that were going to die anyway." She scribbled on a piece of paper even though the rule of office was to use their docuslate for any notes.

"That's very simplistic," Argaret said. "First of all, he lied. Told the public the patch was a stabilizer when it was an accelerator that killed anyone with VMAS."

C.C. piped in. "We have a stabilizer that works. Why wasn't that used?"

"Don't be such a sissy," Gary said. "We can't waste resources or money on people who are on their way out."

"You didn't feel that way about it when your sister contracted VMAS," Argaret said.

"Well, hell, she's my sister," Gary said.

"God, you're dense," Marinda said to Gary.

"Personally, I know Emory pretty well, and it's important to him that we cut back on the population." Adam shifted in his seat, obviously uncomfortable with the whole business.

"Yeah, but it's pretty plain he was targeting people with no connections since they couldn't get the real stabilizer," C.C. said. "People he considers riff raff."

"Well, aren't they?" Marinda was red-faced again. "I say, well done."

"Okay," Adam said. "We're just going over the same ground we've been covering since we started conferencing. Time to make a decision."

"Look at it this way," Argaret said. "It was a nightmare on those streets with people dying all around. Think of the panic it caused. Many died being trampled ... particularly children."

"Emory would love that. The more dead, the better." Marinda said, smirking.

Adam said, "Okay. Let's get a preliminary vote. Remember: Guilty is an automatic death penalty for a crime of this caliber."

There was no hesitation.

Two Guilty.

Two Not Guilty.

Adam let out a deep sigh. He knew if he let Emory Dutton off there would be a huge outcry, especially after the election. The last thing they needed was some kind of active revolution. It was bad enough that he would have to deal with the Defys and the results of the election. He had no doubt—the Defys would no longer be a secret organization.

Still, Adam needed a new liver. Emory had always taken care of the right people; maybe a Medi-Prog CEO replacement would do the same.

No matter what happens, Dutton's never going to keep his position. Better safe than sorry. I need to help the upper class so they believe in me. Yet, help the Defys so they trust me.

"Argaret, C.C., I will vote guilty and break the tie, if we extend leniency."

"What kind of leniency did you have in mind, Adam?"

"Expulsion to the Noncorps."

There was a long moment of silence. C.C. and Aragret each nodded.

"Well, that's it. Tomorrow we will officially inform Emory Dutton of our decision."

* * *

The telelink buzzed. Dutton looked at the window in the communicator.

Adam Fiss.

"Hello, Emory."

Dutton swallowed hard. His ears were ringing.

"Adam. Tell me."

"I'm sorry. It's bad news ... a guilty verdict." There was a long hesitation. "I shouldn't be telling you this before you return to our hearing room, but I wanted to give you a chance to think about things."

"I was hoping ... since you retained your seat, I might have a chance."

"With new members being seated, probably Defy backed people ... well, I can't afford to go against a populist vote." Adam's voice lowered. "I'm sure you understand."

"Why should I understand? You and your idiot members are the ones who should understand. Everything I have done has been for the benefit of our Corporit system. I worked for the benefit of *our* people. You seem to have forgotten about that."

Adam's voice turned to ice. "At least you've avoided the death penalty. Be grateful for that."

Dutton could feel his chest growing tighter and tighter with each breath. "So they won't kill me. What are they going to do to me?"

"Expulsion to the Noncorps."

Dutton saw spots before his eyes as an eruption of rage swelled through his veins. He disconnected the link and stood shaking for several minutes.

He reactivated the telelink.

"Edgar, get to my apartment with the limo. Now!"

* * *

George Potek was watching the election results, screaming cheers at the screen. Every candidate he'd voted for was elected. He knew the new members, had seen their files. They were probably Defys, but it was time to change a few things. Maybe the Defys would do that. He'd thought long and hard about voting for a repeat of Adam Fiss as the Chief Interrogator. But Potek liked the man, didn't want to take a chance on a new CIC chief. Fiss would have to do.

In the middle of watching the returns, his CAPO telelink line, on hold for thirty minutes, automatically returned to service and started going crazy. He punched into line.

#1: Call back time—2115.

"Sir, this is Marshal Number Seventeen reporting with an updated report on Melik and Jin Bacha."

"Proceed," Potek said.

"They have departed from their residence in the Bacha van. Recorded destination: the Organ Harvesters complex."

"Stay with them."

"Yes, sir."

Line#2: Call back time—2125.

"Sir, this is Number Sixteen reporting with an update on surveillance of Doctor Andrew Potter and an unidentified woman. They are traveling in a van registered to Becky Quinn. It appears their destination, although unrecorded, is the Organ Harvesters complex."

"Stay with them."

"Yes, sir."

Line #3: Call back time—2135.

"Sir, this is Marshal Number Eighteen reporting with an update on CEO Emory Dutton, who is traveling in his private limousine."

"Proceed."

"The destination has not been recorded, but it appears the limo is traveling to the edge of Sanfrancorp. Possible destination: the Organ Harvesters complex."

"Continue constant observation."

"Yes, sir."

Why are they all going to that damn building? And Dutton? What the hell is he up to now?

Potek was up and out the door of his apartment.

Chapter 58

ORGAN HARVESTER COMPLEX

Jin had passed out. When she finally awoke, her mind started racing. She should have been screaming in pain. There shouldn't have been a part of her that wasn't in agony, but only her face was hurting. She stared at the opening of her robe as if it belonged to someone else. The whole front of it was soaked with blood—a metallic odor wafted over her.

They must have been on the road a long time, but her sense of time and place was distorted. Every now and then, Melik would reach out and pound her face.

Wisps of memories of Andrew would flip through her head. She didn't want to think about him and the life they could have had. If her hands were free she would use the handle, open the door, and fall on the road as they sped. Maybe it would kill her—at least it would all be over. All she hoped for was a quick death. But she knew Melik wasn't through with her—he thrived on the pain of others. He would make her suffer even more.

She started to drift when he shook her violently.

"We're here, baby doll. We're at the Organ Harvesters complex. You're going to love it. This is our biggest and best client. I know this place inside out and I'm going to show you around."

"Organ ...?"

"Yeah. I'll bet you've never been inside." He laughed. "Some reporter! You probably think this place is some kind of humanitarian project that the Medi-Progs sponsor for the populace—or as they like to say, for the benefit of mankind." He shook her again. "Mankind, not womankind. Get it?"

His voice kept flowing in and out along with a strange ringing in her ears. It had started the last time he punched the side of her face and it hadn't stopped since. She opened her eyes wide and looked over at Melik.

Why did I marry you? Oh, I remember. I thought I loved you. I didn't want to be alone. I've never been more alone than in the last five years ... until Andrew ... Andrew. I'll never see you again.

Tears started trickling down her cheeks. She tried to turn in her seat but her robe ripped away from her skin. She looked down at a fresh spurt of blood seeping through the clotted cloth.

Got to get out of here. Got to get away from him.

They were in front of a huge windowless building. As they circled around to what must have been the back, Melik started whistling one of the songs she particularly hated. It was harsh and had a strange beat that always made her teeth tingle. But her mouth was now too numb to really feel anything. For some strange reason she wanted to laugh at that even though she knew it wasn't really funny.

He stopped whistling, turned off the ignition, and the almost nonexistent sound from the engine died.

* * *

Becky and Tris Quinn each clasped Zoe in a tight hug. Then they reached for Andrew.

"How do you know Melik will take her to Organ Harvesters?" Tris asked.

Zoe saw that both Becky and Tris's faces were sunken, chalk-white, and their eyes were large and filled with fear.

"It's the only place he can really get rid of her without the CAPOs getting involved," Andrew said.

"Oh, my god," Becky said.

Tris grabbed Zoe's hands. "Bring our niece back."

They climbed into the small van and drove off.

Zoe had to talk. Had to hear her own voice, Andrew's voice, or her fear would overwhelm her. "It's a good thing you know how to drive. I've never had a car and I would probably run into a wall."

He was silent for a moment, but when he spoke his voice was so low she had to strain to hear him. "I will kill Melik."

"I'm so sorry."

"There's one thing you will have to settle if anything happens to me, Zoe."

"Don't say that, Andrew. We'll reroute the computer directives in the main board together. We'll search for neural function for the people trapped inside those tanks." Zoe squeezed his hand. "If any of one of them have brain activity within normal limits, we'll try for revival."

"If for some reason I don't make it, you'll have to do it alone, Zoe. I've left you step-by-step instructions. You'll know what to do?"

"And if all of those people in the tanks are into neural death mode?"

"Destroy the place. Its existence is nothing but a nightmare."

"I'll do what needs to be done."

His pocket telelink buzzed. He lifted it out from his jacket. "Hello."

Zoe watched his face closely. A big smile made him look like a little boy. Then he disconnected.

He reached out and squeezed her hand. "That was Argaret Charles. She called about the great outcome of the election—to say that Dutton has been found guilty."

"Well, that's fantastic news on both counts," she said.

"They're going to expel him to the Noncorps."

"What! Why does he get to walk away? He should be executed," she said. "Even that hardly balances what he's done to thousands of people. And Nathan and Seka? It's not fair to them. They lost their lives."

"I know," Andrew said. "I feel the same way, but nothing will bring them back."

"And now the Noncorps will be stuck with him."

"He won't survive even twenty-four hours out on his own."

"Still—"

"Zoe, I can't tell you how proud I am of you. You've gone from someone who wanted no part of the Defy rebellion to a person who helped turn everything around. There's real hope with the fantastic outcome of the election."

"Thanks, Andrew. That means a lot coming from you."

Andrew doused the car lights as they drove up to the Organ Harvesting complex There was barely any illumination around the perimeter. The place seemed to rise out of hell like a dark apparition. Memories of all the years she'd worked in that hopeless environment hit her hard. She fought to stay focused on the present.

"I don't see any vans around here. Maybe they're not here." Zoe covered her mouth. "Oh, my god, where would he take her? How will we find her?"

"Take it easy." He swung the car around, past the Nicola Fountain and the employee park. "Let's circle the building. Don't forget, Melik would enter through a different entrance from the medical staff."

Zoe's heart was racing, her mind spinning with all kinds of crazy scenarios—all of them leading to Jin's death. Her heart sank as they circled the empty lot around the facility. On the far side they saw a van parked and on the driver's door the INSTRUCORP Bacha logo was inscribed in bold letters.

"That's his," Andrew said. "It has the family business logo on it."

Chapter 59

Emory Dutton remembered the times he would ride in this limo to visit his mistress, Taura.

What an amazing bed partner— could fuck my brains out.

Had to cheat on me ... with my own driver.

Well, Taura had her chance. Now she's an organ donor, along with many who thought they were smarter than me. No one stabs me in the back and gets away with it.

No one.

But her lovely face floated before his eyes. He reached for a crystal tumbler, filled it with Scotch. There was no denying it—he missed her.

"How did you get the limo, Edgar?" He let out a bitter grunt. "I'm not supposed to have any privileges like this anymore."

"I just took it, sir."

"Good man!"

The booze wasn't making him high anymore, it didn't even relax him. Tonight, drinking only made him angrier. Right now he wanted to put his fist through the window, or choke Argaret Charles, the CIC member who always criticized him and the Corporit CEOs the most.

Instead, he opened the hidden compartment in the arm rest. He stared down at a gun nestled inside; he'd kept it in case someone tried to kidnap him. There'd been an attempt only once, but Dutton was a fast learner. Now he had this secret protector. It used to tickle his fancy—no one knew it was there, at least not by looking at the plush panel.

Who was he kidding? Maybe there really was no such thing as secrets. After all, everyone now knew about his doctored VMAS stabilizer.

My own fault. What an idiot. Had to tell them, didn't I?

I could have just done it—had a private arrangement. Even Pharmcorp's CEO would have gone along with it. After all, he was still alive with a 'donated' heart, arranged for by me.

No. I had to go with some startup company that did it for practically nothing.

Crimes against humanity?

What the hell does that mean in this world they'd created? Fucking humans can't stop reproducing. They steal each other's air, the very air they all breathe.

Now that's a crime against humanity.

* * *

George Potek sat in the back of his CAPO van, with a marshal on either side of him.

"Take us to the Organ Harvesters complex."

"Yes, sir."

"What the hell are Melik Bacha and his wife doing there at this time of night?" Potek said to the marshal on his left. "That man's a loose cannon, like his sister."

"With all due respect, sir, there's only one reason he's taking his wife there."

Potek looked at the marshal, one who had been with him from the time he was first made commander. The man had known for years what went on in that complex. Probably all of his CAPOs did.

The marshal lowered his voice. "That doesn't bode well for her."

Bet Melik found out about Andrew Potter. Well, at least I won't have that on my conscience. I never reported her activities with Potter to Melik.

And we don't have the Quinns to deal with. That's a good thing for them. I've given them a pass with that meeting they had before the election, but I won't risk anymore cover-ups.

Potek was feeling a lot better since the election outcome. Maybe things would get better.

"I wonder who the unidentified woman is with Potter," Potek said.

"There was no signature reading on her?" asked the marshal on his right.

"Couldn't even get a fix on her," Potek said.

"Sir, Emory Dutton is on the move," the other marshal said, checking his tracker.

The man's a convicted criminal and he's taking off from his home. Dutton can't be running, can he?

Another loose cannon.

Chapter 60

ORGAN HARVESTER COMPLEX
ADMISSIONS

Melik half-dragged, half-lifted Jin as they stepped into what looked like the instrument supply rooms. The walls were a bright white and reflected light bounced off the flat surfaces and made her eyes burn.

A painted sign on the wall said:

INSTRU-CORP—FINE INSTRUMENTS

She saw what seemed like miles and miles of long rectangular tables—they were everywhere. On them was a spread of all kinds of shiny instruments that Melik's company made. Mostly, there were assortments of knives lined up, from very small to huge, hatchet-size.

Melik walked away. It looked like he was doing something to a panel on the wall. He must have been trying disconnect some kind of alarm system—one that had started to blast throughout the room.

Jin was exhausted; her left eye was swollen shut and her right eye kept drooping. It was hard to follow his movements and her focus kept flipping in and out. She turned away when everything was silent again and lay her head on the edge of one of the tables and watched her blood drip from her robe onto the floor.

"Beautiful, isn't it?" Melik returned to her side again. He did a sweep of the room with one hand.

Jin barely heard him. She was wasted and wanted to run, to be anyplace but here, but she couldn't will her body to do anything. She felt like a puppet waiting for strings to move her in some kind of direction so she could function and feel alive again.

When she didn't respond, he tossed her to the floor. She looked up at his face, which had turned dark with anger. He pulled her up, yanked hard on her arm, trying to make her move. She kept falling, and no matter how hard he yanked, whether it was his hands tugging her arms or his fingers pulling her hair, she fell back to the floor.

"So you think this is the end of it? I'll be back with a stretcher; we have plenty of those. The kidneys in your body are going to Marinda. Chew on that for a while."

She watched with numb detachment as he left the room.

Her kidneys were going to be Marinda's. That didn't make sense. Everything was confusing.

She tried to stand, she needed to run away. But her legs gave way and, with her hands tied behind her, there wasn't anything she could do.

Then, as if someone turned on a switch deep within, she was awake with sudden undulating pain that shot from every part of her—burning hot spikes stabbed every inch of her body.

She screamed and tried to crawl, but every time she moved it drove her into a blind frenzy of unrelenting pain.

"Oh, shut up!" Melik said, returning with a gurney. "I wondered when that shot I gave you would wear off. The timing's perfect."

He untied her hands, lifted her, and threw her onto the stretcher.

"Melik, please, please, please stop. Let me go. I won't tell anyone." She screamed, and the words spilled from her mouth. "I can't stand the pain. Please!"

"You won't tell? Of course you won't tell." Then he laughed. "We're going for a ride, Jin."

He bent over and gave her a smile as she tried not to scream out again.

"How many times have I asked you to come and see where I spend so much of my time?"

"Please, Melik! Stop! I couldn't take off time whenever I wanted to. I have a job."

"Not anymore you don't. See how quickly things can change, my little pet. Being my wife wasn't a big enough job for you ... taking care of me wasn't enough for you ... doing what I told you to do, wasn't enough for you."

He rolled her into a huge rotunda. What looked like gigantic fish tanks were everywhere.

All those tubes coming from the ceiling. What are they? What's inside?

"Oh, my god! Melik!" She stared at the tanks. "Are those people?"

This must be where they took my friend, Ethan.

"Why, yes. Those are stupid people, just like you. My daddy used to say, fucked up people who couldn't do what they were told. Dumb, stupid, cows, like you."

"No, no, no!" Her mind went blank, all she could do was yell his name.

"Melik, Melik, Melik."

* * *

The night admissions tech stood decked out in his white coveralls. He gave Melik a nasty sneer.

"Jeez, Melik. What's this bloody mess you've brought me?" The tech ripped open Jin's robe. "She's covered in blood."

"Well, it's not my fault you started her bleeding up again, yanking her robe like that," Melik said.

Melik watched Jin shiver and whimper. Her voice was ragged and almost gone from screaming.

The tech looked up at Melik. "You can go now. I do better when I work alone."

"Is that so?" Melik said. "I don't give a shit what you want. I'm not leaving until I see those kidneys in one of those containers. He pointed to large glass vats. And I want to see Marina Bacha on the ident tag. Get me?"

The tech started washing off the gobs of blood that had seeped all over her body. She started shivering, her arms jumping all over the table.

"Here," Melik said. "Let me hold her down."

"Get your hands off of her. I'm trying to clean her up for surgery and you're contaminating everything with your big, clumsy hands. Your sis is not going to like to see her kidneys infected and useless."

"Okay, okay," Melik said, stepping back.

The tech scrubbed until he'd removed the clotted blood and exposed the open breast bone to navel wound. "Nice technique, but you sure as hell are not a surgeon."

"Ha, ha. Aren't you funny," Melik said. "Get to it. I don't have all night."

"First of all, she's drained off enough blood that she might just up and die. That's not too good, is it?"

"So she dies and you take those kidneys. Big deal."

The tech pulled out his needles and started searching for a vein. It took a while but he finally hit the vessel and attached an IV bag with fluid.

"I just want the kidneys for my sister. I don't care about the rest of her."

"I know what you want, but I'm not losing my job over you just wanting these kidneys. Get it?" The tech pulled out an oxygen mask, attached the tubing to a gadget in the wall. "You want to stay? Fine. But it's going to take some time. Like it or not."

Melik pulled up a chair from the far side of the room and sat down.

Chapter 61

Andrew flipped the van's interior lights off as he and Zoe pulled up to the Organ Harvesters back entrance, next to the Bacha van.

"They must be here," Zoe said.

He reached for the gun resting on the seat between them. Safety off, he tucked it in his back waistband. "I hope I don't have to use this thing."

"It's ready to fire?"

"It is now."

They left the van and headed for the back door to the complex. INSTRU-CORP was scrolled across it. Andrew slid in his ident-card and the door opened.

Inside the room, blinding lights reflected on the walls and the instruments, stopping them in their tracks.

"I recognize these," she said, pointing to the knives on the tables. "I was hoping never to see them again."

"I don't know much about this end of the place. I have no idea where Jin and Melik can be."

"I know," Zoe said. "Follow me."

They edged their way through a maze of corridors, some very narrow, but they finally came to the rotunda.

Andrew said, "When Jin asked me to find Ethan, it was the first time I'd been here in years." He stopped to look into a tank: a shaved-headed woman stared back at him with unseeing eyes.

Zoe read the Ident next to a number on the card. It read: *Taura Missen. Age 26.* The date of the placement was only a short time ago.

"People like her are the reason I needed that info on the control room. She's been stashed here recently." Andrew pointed at the tank. "Some of these individuals might still have cognitive brain activity. We can try to save them."

"I don't know. So many have been stripped of their organs and other parts." She turned away from the tank. "If they have a functioning brain left, they must all be insane by now."

* * *

Emory Dutton continued to bully his driver Edgar, forced him to drive him to the Organ Harvesting Complex, even though it had been specifically declared off limits by the CIC at the beginning of his trial.

"Go around to that entrance over there." When they parked, Dutton stepped out and reached in the back of the van for the large fluid-filled metal container that he'd brought with him.

After using his Ident for admittance, he keyed into the special visitor's elevator to the top floor. They probably hadn't had a chance to change his status qualification. His presence wouldn't set off any alarms—yet.

He stepped away from the elevator and walked to the center. He was now closer to the large mass of bladders that fed nutrients and oxygen to the people in the tanks via a massive tubing system. He set the heavy container down and stretched his shoulder. Sweat ran down his back and his heart was pounding in his throat.

* * *

"Pull up behind that limo," Potek said to the driver. "You men stay here until I call for you."

"Yes, sir," they said in unison.

Potek walked up to the limo driver's window and tapped. It slid down. Potek recognized the driver.

"What can I do for you, commander?"

"Edgar, do you know why Mr. Dutton had you drive him here tonight?"

"No, sir. I just do as I'm told."

Potek signaled to the men in the car and they were with him in a moment.

"You," he said, pointing to one of the marshals, "go to admissions, see if they can check out Dutton's whereabouts." He pointed to the others. "All of you stay with me. Let's go in here. Have your guns at the ready."

"Yes, sir," the group answered as one.

* * *

Zoe and Andrew left the rotunda—she led them down a very narrow corridor where they had to stoop to keep from banging their heads. Every step seemed to release an overwhelming stink of death. Ahead, there were bright lights, they heard loud voices.

"I don't want her to have anything. I want her to suffer. Do you hear me? Suffer!"

"If she moves around on the table, I guarantee those kidneys you want so badly for your sister will be lacerated and totally useless."

"Melik, please don't do this. I'm begging you."

"I warned you, my little blossom flower, told you I would make you suffer for sleeping with that robot doctor. Now you know I'm a man of my word. Bitch!"

"Are we doing this, or aren't we?"

"Okay, give it to her. But do it fast. I can't spend all night here."

Zoe and Andrew looked at each other with shock, then burst into the room. Andrew went for Melik, reached out and grabbed him by the neck.

The technician was already dosing Jin. Her eyes were shut. The technician looked at Zoe. His mouth dropped open when she snatched a knife from a surgical stand and held it out ready to stab him.

"Hey, I'm just a drone. Don't blame it on me."

Zoe hesitated and he reached out and almost grabbed her. She stabbed him in the arm.

He screamed at the top of his lungs. "That hurts like hell!"

"Do that again and I'll cut your heart out."

"Okay. Okay!"

Andrew and Melik were rolling on the floor, Melik under Andrew, the gun slipping out of his waistband. Zoe grabbed it.

"I should have killed you when I had you, you bastard," Melik ranted. He chopped Andrew across the throat, quickly stood while Andrew gagged.

Melik picked up a chair, ready to smash it down on Andrew.

"Put that down," Zoe yelled. "Put it down now!"

She held the gun out in front of her and stood where she could shoot either Melik or the technician.

Melik looked at her, a sneer crossed his face.

As he brought the chair down, Zoe shot him in the chest. His shirt blossomed with a spread of blood and his knees gave way. The chair glanced off of Andrew.

A look of surprise crossed Melik's face before he hit the floor—dead.

One of Potek's marshals walked into the room, his gun at the ready.

"What's going on here?"

* * *

George Potek couldn't understand why Dutton had come to Organ Harvesters.

What's the ass doing here of all places? What the hell is he up to?

It hit him in a flash.

He headed for the back stairs, marshals following close at his heels.

* * *

Dutton scouted around until he found tubing in a supply closet. It wasn't heavy, but it was awkward. He dragged it to the edge of the landing, hoisted it with one hand and picked up the container with the other.

He stepped onto the narrow walkway. It was difficult while balancing with things in both hands. He tried not to look down to the bottom of the ten stories. It would be a long way to fall.

298

Chills raced up and down his spine, made him feel weak. His legs were wobbly and he had the strangest feeling that the eyes of the specimens in the tanks were following his every move. Waves of hatred surrounded him.

Yes, all those specimens wanted him to fall.

He reached the ledge surrounding the huge bladders that were the massive providers, the heart of the life support system.

Nutrients, fluids, and oxygen, all flowed down from here into every tank and each occupant's life depended on these tubes. He carefully set the container down on the narrow ledge and pulled a knife from his pocket. He stabbed through each bladder and forced a section of tubing inside. For a moment he stood transfixed, watching the leakage drip around the tubes down into the rotunda.

The sound of someone shouting brought him to the moment.

He opened the container and pulled out a small retracted spout and poured the fluid into the tubes. He knew it was infusing all the specimens in the tanks and even from high above, he could hear not only the specimens in the tanks thrashing, but the warning alarms screeching.

* * *

"Stop it!" Potek yelled out to Dutton. "You hear me. Stop it!"

Dutton turned toward the voice.

"Potek, is that you?"

"Yes, sir. It's me." He watched Dutton pull a long thick wooden match from his pocket.

"Not so stupid after all."

"Come back off the ledge."

"I don't think so, Potek."

"Why are you doing this?"

"So, you're still the same old idiot you've always been. Dumber than dumb."

"That's not an answer, sir."

"Like always, it needs to be spelled out for you."

"Come down from there, sir."

"Don't you get it?" Dutton yelled. "You stupid fool!" He waved an arm. "This was going to be my legacy. Mine! My gift to all the Corporits that deserved to live. For all the people who run this world. *They* deserve to live forever, not the drones of this world."

"Sir—"

"Send me to the Noncorps! Noncorps are fools. I'm not a fool. Noncorps are losers. I'm not a loser."

Without another word, he held a tube from the nutrient pouch, lit the match, and watched the flame whoosh into the huge bladder and down the tubes.

All the tanks around them and in the rotunda exploded—flames shot out everywhere.

The last sight he had of Dutton was in the center of flames burning the platform around him. When Potek reached the stairs, there was a shot.

Dutton wasn't into suffering.

Potek and the marshals raced down the stairs.

* * *

Zoe, Andrew, Jin, and others were already outside of the complex when Potek and his marshals ran out. Most raced away into the Nicola fountain park next to the facility—Zoe ran and hid in the van.

The limo driver and the CAPO van were already there.

When the interior of the complex exploded, it was like a celebration of fireworks shooting up into the sky.

Chapter 62

THE DOMES

Zoe and Storm were wrapped in each other's arms. They lay on the soft mossy ground and stared at a rare sight—a pollution free sky filled with a universe of stars.

Wolf sat on his haunches next to Zoe. He hadn't left her side since she returned three days ago, but neither had Storm.

"And Jin is no longer a cub reporter for News-Div," Zoe said. "I guess everybody felt she'd earned her stripes. She was very brave getting the news out to help the Defys. And, she paid the price. She was horribly beaten by Melik and lost an eye. For a while, it was touch and go whether she would even survive."

"The new CIC elections? Do you think the results will change anything?" Storm's fingers slid up and down her arms.

"I hope so. Tris Quinn has totally come out of retirement. He and Becky are working to restructure the entire health care system."

"And the new CIC?" Storm asked, his voice trailing off.

"They've started flexing their muscles," Zoe said. "All global Organ Harvesters' satellites will now come under the Quinn Foundation's strict review and recommendations. I think it's safe to say, those tanks are a thing of the past."

She wrapped her arms around his waist and they kissed for a long time.

"Andrew offered to help in any way he could, too. He's still upset that because of Emory Dutton, we couldn't save any of the people trapped in the tanks. It was very important to him."

Storm raised an eyebrow, "Do you really believe it was possible?"

Zoe leaned back into his chest. "No. I don't think we could have saved any of them. But I admire him for wanting to try."

"And how do you feel?" he asked

"Very lucky. In the commotion of the tanks and the complex exploding, I was able to sneak back to the van before the head CAPO could focus on my 'kill on sight' face."

"Yes, you are a lucky woman ... and very brave."

"And yet, I'm still sad. Nathan Quinn and Seka Joraine are gone—no matter what I do." Tears ran down her cheek and when she looked at Storm, tears were running down his cheeks, too.

* * *

Zoe was at the school dormitory—special permission to interrupt Laya's adjustment program had been given by the Children's Council.

She'd promised to tell Laya a fairy tale before she went to sleep.

"I think I'm really going to like it here, Mom."

Zoe missed being called Mommy, but she could see her daughter had blossomed and matured in a short time in the domes.

"I want you to be happy."

Laya lay back, snuggled up close to her mother. "Tell me a story, please."

Zoe ran her fingers through her daughter's hair and kissed her cheek. She began:

"Once upon a time there was a beautiful planet called Earth. All the people who lived there loved all the animals and they treasured Mother Nature ..."

The End

Acknowledgements

The Group: Margaret (Peggy) Lucke, Shelley Singer, Nicola Trwst, Judith Yamamoto, and, above all, J. J. Lamb, who is always there for me, through the good, the bad, and the ugly and still loves me. Hard to believe.

Web and cover design guru, Sue Trowbridge.

Many thanks to Marcia Muller and Bill Pronzini, MWA Grand Masters and especially grand, supportive friends; to our other supportive writer-friends: Rita Lakin, Shelley Singer, Margaret and Charlie Lucke, Jaki Girdner, Greg Booi, Ellen Kirschman, Ken Gwin, Tree Gee, Julie Smith, Barbara Yeninas And to our loyal reader-friends Regina and Bill Thomas, Patti Harais, Tris Donlevy,

My medical pals, Gabe Farkas and Katie Velick, Betty Hannigan, Sydney Yamashita—for all the medical conversations that tickled my brain cells over many years.

So many others—friends, readers, too many to mention, but you know who you are. Please believe I'm grateful to every one of you.

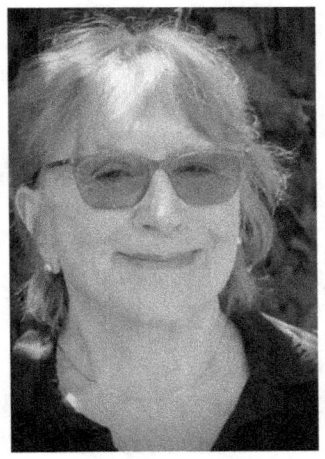

About the Author

Bette Golden Lamb, unmistakably from The Bronx, can usually be found at her desk writing, or in her studio playing with clay, or in her garden tending to some 50 rose bushes. There are times, though, when she sets all of this aside and sneaks off to the movies.

An RN, she is the author or co-author of almost a dozen novels, mostly medical thrillers, with a smattering of near-future and suspense-adventure books thrown in for good measure. Her most recent near-future medical novel is prize-winning *The Organ Harvesters.*

She is also a professional ceramist, sculptor, and artist, whose award-winning creations appear in regional, national and international shows and exhibitions, and are shown in galleries.

Born in New York, her peripatetic career has taken her to live in Virginia, New Mexico, California, back to New York, Nevada, and back to California, where she now lives with her co-author husband, J. J.